Medical Swahili

Phrasebook and Glossary

1

first edition 2013

ISBN is 1494464659
EAN-13 is 978-1494464653

by A.H.Zemback

Contents

Introduction/demographics

Introduction/ demographics	English	Swahili
	How are you?	Habari yako?
	Good morning, good afternoon, good evening	Habari ya asubuhi, habari za mchana, mema jioni.
	My name is ...	Jina langu ni...
	I am a... (1)nurse, (2)doctor, (3)social worker, (4)dentist, (5)eye doctor, (6)surgeon, (7) physical therapist	Mimi ni...(1)mwuguzi, (2)daktari, (3)msaidizi wa tiba(4)daktari wa meno,(5) daktari wa macho (6) daktari wa upsuaji (7) kimwili mtaalamu
	What is your name?	Jina lako ni nani?
	Can you write it in English?	Je, unaweza kuliandika kwa Kiingereza?
	I am pleased to meet you.	Nimefurahi kukutana nawe.
	Please write your name here.	Andika jina lako hana, tafadhali.
	Do you speak English?	Unasema kiingereza?
	I don't speak Swahili.	Sisemi kiswahili.
	Say that one more time, please.	Tafadhali kurudia kwamba.
	I don't understand.	Siselewi.
	Can you speak slowly, please?	Sema polepole, tafadhali.
	Come with me.	Fuatana nami, tafadhali.
	Sit down, please.	Kaa chini, tafadhali.
	What province do you live in?	Manaisha wilasani gani?
	What is your address?	Unakaa wapi?
	What is your telephone number?	Kile ni nambari yako ya simu?
	Do you have an I.D?	Una kitambulisho?
	Can you give us the name and telephone number or address of someone to be contacted?	Unaweza kutupa jina na namba ya simu au anwani ya mtu ambaye tunaweza kumpa habari zako?
	Are you married?	Ulishaka owa (for male)? Ulishaka wolewa (for female)
	What is your age?	Una umri wa miaka mingapi?

Chief Complaint

Chief complaint	English	Swahili
	chief complaint	jambo ambalo mgonjwa analalamikia
	What is your health concern today?	Uko na tatizo gani?
	When did this problem start?	Hiyi shida ilianza lini?
	How many days have you been feeling ill?	Umekuwa na ugonjwa kwa siku ngapi?
	Have you had an accident?	Ulikuwa kwenya ajali?
	Is this injury from a landmine?	Jeraha hili linatokana na bomu la kuzika ardhini?
	Were you shot with a gun?	Ulipigwa risasi?
	Is this from a machete?	Hii inatoka kwa panga?
	Is this from a car accident?	Hii inatoka kwa ajali ya gari?
	Did you lose consciousness after this happened?	Ulipoteza fahamu baada ya hii kufanyika?
	Did you lose a lot of blood before coming here?	Unapoteza dau zaidi ya kiasi hiki?
	What medicine have you taken?	Nini dawa hamajapata?
	Do you have any pain?	Una umwa yoyote?
	When did the pain start (use the calendar to show me)?	Ilianza lini? (onyesha kwenya kalenda na saa)
	How many days have you had the pain?	Umekuwa na maumivu kwa siku ngapi?
	What is your level of pain ? 0= no pain, 10 = severe pain	Waywe na uma kidogo kama mwingi? 0 = pana uma, 10 = uma kabisa
	Hold up the number of fingers.	Shika juu namba ya vidole vyako.
	Is the pain severe?	Jee maumivu ni mengi sana?
	Is the pain sharp or dull?	Hea ni maumivu makali au yaliyofifia?
	Is your pain burning?	Una maumivu kiwasho?
	Is your pain cramping?	Hea ni maumivu yaneochoma?
	Is the pain constant...?	Hea ni maumivu ya daima?
	or does it come and go?	Au yanakwenda na kurudi?

Chief complaint	English	Swahili
	Does the pain go to your back?	Maumivu yanaenda mgongoni?
	Touch the spot where it hurts with one finger.	Tia mkono kwenye unaumizwa.
	What makes it better?	Ni nini inapunguza maumivu?
	What makes it worse?	Ni nin inazidisha?
	When do you get the pain...	Wakati gani unasikia unaumizwa...
	at night, before meals, after meals?	usiku, kabla hujakula ao kisha kula?
	Have you been in the hospital before?	Umekuwa katika hospitali kabla ya?
	What were you treated for?	Nini tiba gani kupokea katika hospitali?

Common Complaints

Common complaints	English	Swahili
	My lower back hurts.	Mgongo yangu imeumwa (ina maumivu).
	My neck is stiff.	Shingo yangu ina ugumu. (Shingo yangu ni ngumu.
	I have a sore throat.	Niko namaumivu ndani ya shingo.
	I have a fever	Niko na homa.
	I have night sweats.	Niko natoka jasho usiku.
	It hurts when I swallow.	Nina umwa wakati ya kumeza.
	I have an earache.	Nina maumivu ku sikio.
	I have poor vision.	Siko naona vuzuri.
	I have a toothache.	Lino (jino) iko nani luma.
	My tooth is loose.	Lino (jino) yangu iko na tingizika.
	My dentures are loose and my gums hurt.	Meno yangu ziko zina tingizika na nyama ya meno ikona(l)uma.
	My filling fell out.	Kfuniko ya jino langu ime anguka. (Kizibo ya jinno langu ime anguka)
	My gums bleed when I brush my teeth.	Nyama yamenno yangu iko natowa damu wakati mina sukula meno na mswaki.
	I have shoulder pain.	Nina maumivu ku bega.
	I have elbow pain.	Nina maumivu ku kisugudi (ku mkono).
	I have wrist pain	Nina maumivu ku kiganja (mkono). Kiganja (mkono) iko naniuma.
	I have knee pain.	Nina maumivu ku goti.
	I have ankle pain.	Nina maumivu ku (kifundo cha) mguu.
	I am dizzy.	Nina kizunguzungu.
	I am very nervous.	Nimesirika (Ninasirika) sana.
	I can't sleep.	Si wezi kulala.
	I am tired.	Nimechoka. (Ninachoka)
	I have chest pain.	Nina maumivu ku (ya) kifua.
	My heart beats very fast.	Roho (Moyo) yangu iko napiga mbiyo mbiyo.
	I have a headache.	Nina maumivu ku(ya) kichwa.
	I have trouble breathing.	Nina shindwa kupumuwa.
	I am short of breath at night.	Niko nashindwa kupumuwa usiku.

Common complaints	English	Swahili
	I am short of breath with exertion.	Niko nashindwa kupumuwa wakati natumiya nguvu. (wakati ya mazoezi).
	I have to sleep sitting up.	Nina lala wima.
	I am coughing a lot.	Niko nakohowa sana.
	It hurts when I cough.	Nina maumivu wakati nina kohowa. Nasikiya maumivu wakati nina kohowa.
	I have not had a menstrual cycle for ... months.	Miezi...sipati (sioni) siku ya mwezi (hedhi)/Sipati (sioni) siku ya mwezi imepita miezi...
	I think I am pregnant.	Ninawaza kama niko na mimba (mjamzito).
	I have morning sickness.	Niko na ugonjwa wa asubuyi (kutapika kwa mimba).
	I am pregnant	Niko na mimba/niko mjamzito.
	I have pain during my menstrual period.	Wakati wasiku zangu ya mwezi nasikiyaka maumivu.
	I have a vaginal infection.	Nina maambukizi ya uke.
	I am on a birth control pill.	Niko na shukua kidonge ya kuzuwiya uzazi. (Mimi niko kwenye kidonge kuzuwiya uzazi)
	I have a stomach ache.	Nina maumivu ku tumbo.
	I cannot eat.	Siwezi kula.
	I have heartburn.	Nina kiungulia.
	I am nauseated.	Nina kichefuchefu. (Nataka kutapika.)
	I have been vomiting.	Nilikuwa na tapika. (Nina tapika.)
	I have been vomiting worms.	Nilikuwa na tapika manyoka.
	I have indigestion.	Nina kiungulia. (Nina vimbiwa tumbo).
	I have no appetite.	Sina njaa. Siko na hamu ya kula (ya chakula).
	I have diarrhea	Niko na endesha (Niko na hara).
	I am suffering from constipation.	Sipati choo kuu. Ninaumwa na kuziba choo (choo yabisi).
	I have blood in my stool.	Nina damu katika mavi.
	My stools are light colored.	Mavi yangu ina rangi nyeupe/ rangi ya mwangaa.
	I get up at night to urinate.	Nina amuka usiku kukojoa (kukoyola). (Mimi na amka usiku kukojoa.)
	My urine is cloudy.	Mikoyo yangu ni chafu (aitakate). (Mkojo wangu ni chafu.)

Common complaints	English	Swahili
	I have bloody urine.	Nina mkojo wa damu. Mikoyo (mkojo) yangu ni ya damu.
	I have pain with urination.	Nina maumivu wakati na kojoa. (Sa niko nakojoa niko na sikiya maumivu.)
	I feel sick.	Na sikia ungonjwa.
	I feel weak.	Siko na sikiya nguvu.
	I have sprained my...	Nina teuka ku.../Nina shtuko...
	I have pain here.	Niko na maumivu apa.
	I think I broke my arm.	Nafikiri (nina waza) nimevunjika mkono.
	I think I broke my leg.	Nafikiri (nina waza) nimevunjika mguu..
	I have a rash.	Niko na upele. Nina upele.
	I have a boil.	Niko na jipu.
	I have a burn.	Ngozi yangu ime chomwa. Nina ungua.
	I have a wound.	Nina kidonda.
	I am injured.	Nina jeraha.
	I am limping.	Niko kilema.
	He hurt his head.	Ame ji ngonga kichwa. Yeye kugeruhiwa kichwa chake.
	He is unconscious.	Ana poteza ufahamu. Ana poteza akili.
	He is bleeding a lot.	Yeye utokwa na damu nyingi. Iko na tokwa damu mingi.
	He has a broken bone.	Iko namufupa yakuvunjika.
	My baby nurses well.	Mtoto wangu ananyonya (iko na nyonya) vizuri.
	My baby suckles poorly.	Mtoto wangu aiko ananyonya muzuri.
	I don't have enough (breast) milk.	Sina maziwa ya mama ya kutosha. Sina maziwa ya kutosha mu kifua.
	My nipples are cracked.	Vilembwa vya titi zangu ni kavu na kupasuka. Chongo yama ziba yangu iko na kauka na ku pasuka.
	I need a breast pump so I can get milk for the baby.	Nina haja ya pampu ya matiti (liziba) ili ni weze kupata maziwa ya mtoto.

9

Past Medical & Surgical History; list of diseases

Past Medical and Surgical History	English	Swahili
	Are you being treated for any chronic health problem?	Avete una storia di qualsiasi problema di salute cronico?
	Do you have a history of:	Una mojawapo ya yoyote ya magonjwa yafuateo? (Jee anagonjwa ka sawa vifitaoyo...)
	AIDS	ukimwi
	anemia	upungufu wa damu
	arthritis	ugonjwa wa baridi yabisi
	asthma	pumu
	bronchitis	mkamba
	cancer	kansa
	chicken pox	tetekuwanga
	cholera	kipindupindu
	common cold; viral uri	mafua
	congestive heart failure	shtuko la moyo
	depression	huzuni
	diabetes mellitus	ungonjwa ya kisukari
	diphtheria	dondakoo
	eczema	ukurutu
	epilepsy	kifafa
	gonorrhea	kisonono
	heart murmur	uvumi wa moyo
	heart problems	matatizo ya moyo
	hepatitis	homa ya manjano (ugonjwa ya maini)
	herpes simplex	manawa
	hypertension	umuvuduko w'amaraso ukabije
	insect bite	kuumwa vibaya na mdudu
	hepatitis	ugonjwa wa maini
	jaundice	homa ya nyongo ya manjano
	malaria	malaria; homa ya mbu
	measles	surua
	mumps	matubwitubwi; perema
	nervous condition	kurukwa na akili
	paratyphoid fever	homa ya matumbo
	peritonsillar abscess	jipu la kifuko

Past Medical and Surgical History	English	Swahili
	pneumonia	mkamba; kamata
	polio	polio, ugonjwa wa kupooza
	rabies	kalab
	ringworm	choa
	scabies (also used for skin rash)	upele
	scarlet fever	homa ya vipele vyekundu
	schistosomiasis	kichocho
	scurvy	ugonjwa wa ukosefu wa vitamini C
	stroke	ugonjwa wa bungo
	syphilis	kaswende; sekeneko
	tapeworm	maambukizo ya tegu; tegu
	thyroid disease	ugonjwa wa tezi ya kikoromeo
	tonsillitis	uvimbemchu ngu wa kifuko
	tuberculosis	kifua kikuu
	typhoid fever	homa ya matumbo
	warts	madutu
	tuberculosis	kifua kikuu
	whooping cough (pertussis)	kifaduro
	worms (roundworm)	minyoo
	yellow fever	homa wa manjano
	Do you know what HIV means?	Unajua ninamaanish a nin na manenyo virusi vya ukimwi?
	Are you infected with HIV ?	Umeambukiz wa na virusi vya ukimwi?
	You need a blood test to check for HIV.	Unahitaji uchunguzi wa damu kwa virusi vya ukimwi.
	HIV/AIDS	agakoko gotera sida (ukimwi)
	Date starting ARV?	Tarche ulianza tumia dawa ya kupunzuzu maumivu?
	Date and value of last CD4?	Tarch na kimo za CD4?
	Do you have a vaccination record?	Je, una rekodi ya chanjo?
	Have you have pneumonia or meningitis?	Ulishaka gonjwa kamata meningite?
	Have you had surgery in the past?	Umekua umepasuliwa?
	What surgery was done?	Baliku pasula nini?
	What year was the surgery done?	Mwaka gani ulipasuliwa?

Family/social history

Family/social history	English	Swahili
	Is your mother living?	Mama wako angali hai?
	Is your father living?	Baba yako angali hai?
	What did your father/mother die from?	Baba yako/mama yako alikufaka na nini? Ni nini iliuwa baba/ mama yako?
	Do your brothers/sisters have health problems?	Wa kaka/wa dada zako wiko na afyia nzuri? Kaka/dada zako wana magonjwa?
	Do you have any children?	Una watoto wowote?
	What is your religion?	Dini yako ni nini?
	Do you drink alcohol?	Unakunywaka pombe? Unatumiya pombe?
	How many drinks per day?	Unakunywaka marangapi ku siku?
	Do you drink alcohol every day?	Unakunywaka pombe kila siku?
	Do you smoke cigarettes?	Unavuta tumbaku?
	How many cigarettes per day?	Unavuta pakiti ngapi za sigara kwa siku?
	What kind of work do you do?	Kazi yako ni nini?

Medications/allergies

Medications/ allergies	English	Swahili
	I am allergic to...	Mimi ni mzio wa dawa hii...
	Have you had reactions to medications?	Una athari zozote mbea kutokana na dawa?
	What is the name of the medication that you had the reaction to?	Jina la dawa ineosababisha athari mbea ni nini?
	Are you allergic to any medicine?	Kuna dawa ambalo halipatani vizuri na mwili wako?
	Do you take (modern) medication at home?	Unameeza dawa ukiva nyumbani?
	Which medication?	Ambayo dawa?
	Have you taken traditional medication?	Unamadawa mimgine unaowatumia au tiba ya kienyeji?
	Are you taking Bactrim?	Uko unakunyuri bactrim?
	I want to see the medication bottle.	Naitaji cupa ya dawa.

Review of systems: lymph, bone, blood

Review of systems: lymph, bone, blood	English	Swahili
	Do you have skin problems?	Unamumivu ya ngozi ya muili?
	Do you have a rash?	Una vipele ngozini?
	Do you have any blisters or sores?	Una malengelenge?
	Do you have any problems with dry skin?	Una kuongeza ya ngozi?
	Have you had lice?	Umekuwa na chawa (kipwepwe)?
	Have you been bitten by ticks?	Umekuwa kuumwa na kupe?
	Have you seen any rats in your home?	Umeona panya katika nymbo yako?
	Were you bitten by a dog or another animal?	Umekuwa kuumwa mbwa au mnyama mwingine?
	Do you have lymph node enlargement or pain?	Una limfu nodi uvimbe?
	Do you have bone pain?	Uko na maumivu ya mifupa?
	Do you have joint pain?	Uko na maumivu mumaunganiyo (maunganishio)?
	Do you have joint swelling?	Jee maungamishiyo yako inavimbaka? Maunganiyo yako ina vimba?
	Do you have muscle pain?	Una maumivu katika musuli?
	Where is the muscle pain?	Maumivu ya musuli yako wapi?
	Do you have pain in the back or the neck?	Una maumivu ya mgongo au shingo ?
	Have you ever had a blood transfusion?	Umekuwa na kuongezewa damu?
	Do you have bleeding problems?	Unashida ya kuvuya?
	Do you have bleeding from anywhere?	Una kutoka damu mahali popote
	Do you urinate frequently?	Una kojowa ninyi? (Unakojawa kojowa?)
	Are you very thirsty?	Una kiu saazote?
	Have you lost weight?	Jee umekonda? (Ume pungua uzito?)
	Is the ankle pain so severe you cannot walk on it?	Ni maumivu ya kifundo cha mguu hivyo kali huwezi kutembea?

14

Review of systems: lymph, bone, blood	English	Swahili
	Does your knee give way?	Goti lako ime cheza/ime toka nje? (Goti lako ina tingizikaka?)
	Do you feel pain when you move your shoulder?	Ukonasikiya maumivu wakati unatingiza bega lako?
	Have you had any broken bones?	Umewahi kuvunjika mifupa?
	What bones were broken?	Umevunja mifupa gani?

Review of systems: HEENT

Review of systems: HEENT	English	Swahili
	Have you suffered from a head trauma in the past?	Jee kuko wakati uligonjwa kichanwani?
	Do you have dizziness?	Una kizunguzungu?
	Have you blacked-out?	Wewe kupoteza fahamu?(Ulipoteza ufaanu?)
	Do you have vision problems?	Unamatatizi ya kuona?
	Is your vision good in both eyes?	Unaona vizuri katika macho yote?
	Which eye is problematic?	Jicho gani lina tatizo jipya?
	Do you have vision loss?	Una maono ya chini?
	Do you have double vision?	Una maona mara mbili? Una ona kitu/mtu mara mbili?
	Do you have pain in bright light?	Una mauvmivu wakati unaangaliya mwangaza (nuru nyingi)?
	Do you have spots in front of your eyes?	Je, unaweza kuona matangazo mbele ya macho yako?
	Do you have blurred vision?	Una kiwaa?
	Do you have pain in your eyes?	Una maumivu yoyote machoni mwako?
	Do you wear glasses?	Unavaa miwani ya sahihisho?
	Do you use contact lenses?	Unatumia lenzi za plastiki?
	Can you hear well?	Unasikia vizuri?
	Do you have hearing problems?	Unamatatizi ya kisikia?
	Which ear is effected?	Una tatizo na ambayo sikio?
	Do you have pain in your ears?	Una mauvmivu ya sikio?
	Do you have drainage from your ears?	Unatokwa usaha ya sikio?
	Do you have hearing loss in only one ear?	Wala wewe huna kusikia kwenye sikio moja?
	Do you have buzzing in the ears?	Je, wanakabiliwa na mvumo sikioni?
	Do you have nosebleeds?	Je unatokwa damu mu mapuwa?
	Do you have bleeding gums?	Unatokwa damu mu masini?
	Do you have ulcers in your mouth?	Una vidonda vya mdomo?
	Do you have a toothache?	Je uko na umivu ya meno?

Review of systems: HEENT	English	Swahili
	Do you have a broken tooth?	Ni jino yako kuvunjwa?
	Do you have lumps or swelling in your mouth?	Una uvimbe katika mdomo wako?
	Do you have hoarseness (a change in your voice)?	Una uchakacho?
	Do you have a sore throat?	Jee unauremiyaka ku mulibu? (Una maumivu ya koo?)
	Do you have neck stiffness?	Jee uko na maumivu shingoni?

Review of systems:Respiratory/cardiac

Review of systems: respiratory/cardiac	English	Swahili
	Are you short of breath?	Unakatika pumzi?(Una shida ya kupumua?)
	Do you have difficulty breathing when you lay down?	Kuko wakati unakaa ili upumuwe?
	Do you have pain when you take a deep breath?	Unavmia wakati unapupua sana?
	Do you have wheezing?	Je, una sauti mwunzi wakati wa kupumua
	Do you have a cough?	Unakohoa?
	How long have you had the cough?	Ni tangu wakati gani uko unakohowa? Ni mda gani uko unakohowa?
	Do you cough up phlegm?	Ukonatosha ile buchafu ya kikohozi?
	Do you have a lot of sputum?	Uko unatema kikoozi mara na mara?
	Do you have bloody sputum?	Unatema damu?
	What color is your sputum.	Utatema kikoozi ya langi gani?
	Have you had tuberculosis?	Kuna wakati uligonjwa ugonjwa wa kifua kikuu? Ulishaka gonjwa kifua kikuu (ama tuberculose)?
	Where did you receive treatment?	Ni wapi wewe ulipata matibabu? Ni wapi ulipata matunzo?
	How many months did you take the medication?	Ni mwezi ngapi ulichukua dawa? Ni mwezi ngapi uli fanya ukonakunywa (ukonachukua) dawa?
	Do you have chest pain?	Uko na maumivu ya kifua?
	Do you have pain that radiates from your chest to your left arm?	Una maumivu kutoka kifua chako kuinguia mkononi wa kushoto?
	Do you sweat when you have this chest pain?	Unatoka jasho ukiwa na maumivu ya kifua?
	Do you have palpitations?	Una kipapa cha moyo?
	Do you have leg edema?	Una mguu uvimbe?
	Do you have weakness?	Unajisikia dhaifu?

18

Review of systems: GI/GU

Review of systems: GI/GU	English	Swahili
	Do you have abdominal pain?	Unasikia tumba inauma? (Je, una maumivu ya tumbo?)
	Do you have abdominal pain after you eat?	Je, una maumivu ya tumbo baada ya kula?
	When did this problem start?	Hiyi shida ilianza lini?
	Has it been weeks, months, years?	Jee kunapita ma juma miezi au myaka?
	Are you in pain now?	Una maumivu sasa hivi?
	Touch the spot where you have pain with one finger.	Tia mkono kwenye unaumizwa.
	Does it hurt all the time?	Unaumiva wakati wote?
	Does the pain come and go?	Au yanakwenda na kurudi?
	Is the pain better than yesterday?	Jee maumivu inazidi kuliko jana?
	Do you have fever?	Umepatwa na homa?
	How many days have you had a fever?	Umekuwa na homa kwa siku ngapi?
	Do you have chills?	Umepatwa na vipapa (baridi)?
	Do you have night sweats?	Una kutokwa jasho usiku?
	Have you lost your appetite?	Unapoteza hamu ya kula?
	Have you vomited?	Umeshatapika?
	Is your vomit bloody or black?	Kuna damu au rangi nyeusi yoyote katika matapishi yako?
	Have you vomited blood?	Je, kuna damu katika matapishi yako?
	Do you have nausea?	Umepatwa na kichefuchefu?
	Did the nausea start today?	Kichefuchefu kilianza leo?
	How many days have you been nauseated?	Wewe kuwa na kichefuchefu kwa jinsi wengi siku?
	Did you have a bowel movement today?	Je, ulipata choo kubwa leo?
	When was your last stool?	Ulienda choo kikubwa lini kwa mara ya mwisho?
	Are you constipated?	Unafunga choo?
	Can you pass gas?	Unapita shuzi?
	Do you have diarrhea?	Unaharisha yoyote?
	How many times per day?	Marangapi kwa siku?
	Have you passed any black stools?	Cho ako likua hiko mausi kama apana?

19

Review of systems: GI/GU	English	Swahili
	What color is your stool...1) red 2) yellow 3) green 4) black?	Umeharisha rangi gani...1) ni nyekundu 2) ni manjano 3) ni kijani 4) ni nyeusi?
	Do you have anal itching?	Je, una kuwasha katika njia ya haja kubwa?
	Do you have pain with swallowing?	Uko na wumivu kwa kumeza?
	Do you have difficulty swallowing?	Unamatatizi ya kumeza?
	Do you have a burning pain in your stomach?	Unawakaa mu tumbo?
	Are you hungry?	Una njaa?
	When did you last eat?	Ulikula mara ya mwisho lini?
	Have you seen worms in your stools? (Do you have worms?)	Una minyoo?
	Have you had a gastroscopy?	Kuko wakati ulipimwa tumboni kwa kuangalia ndani?
	Do you have pain when you urinate?	Una maumivu yoyote unapokojoa?
	Do you have a burning sensation when you urinate?	Inachoma unapokojoa?
	Do you have penile discharge?	Una usaha uume yako?
	Do you have a sore on your penis?	Je, una mboo kidonda?
	Do you have dark urine?	Una mkojo mweusi?
	What does your urine look like?	Elezea mkojo wako rangi?
	Is your urine cloudy?	Ni mkojo wako machafu?
	Do you have sharp pains in your back where the last rib meets the spine?	Je, una maumivu ya mgongo wako wapi ubavu wa kumi na mbili hukutana mgongo?
	Does the pain go to your scrotum?	Maumivu yanaenda pumbuni?
	Do you have difficulty staring to urinate?	Ni vigumu kukojoa? (Una matatizo kuanza kukojoa?)
	Do you have dribbling after you finish?	Je, una mkojo piga chenga baada ya kumaliza kukojoa?
	How often do you urinate at night?	Unakojoa mara ngapi usku?
	Do you have the urge to urinate but can't pass any urine?	Una hamu ya kukojoa lakini huwezi kupitisha mkojo?
	Is the urine stream slow?	Je kukojoa polepole?
	Have you urinated today?	Umekojoa leo?

Review of systems: GI/GU	English	Swahili
	Does your bladder feel full?	Kibofu chako kinahisi kama kimejaa?
	Do you leak urine when you cough or sneeze?	Ni wewe sasiojizuia ya mkojo kama wewe kuchafya.
	Do you have blood in the urine?	Kuna damu katika mkojo?
	Have you every passed a kidney stone?	Umekufikia kutowa kijiwe la figo?
	Do you have incontinence?	Ni wewe sasiojizuia ya mkojo?

Review of systems: Women's Health

Review of systems:Women's Health	English	Swahili
	Have you noticed any breast lumps?	Uko na shida kua matiti?
	Do you have nipple discharge?	Kuna maziwa yanakoka kwa mziba yako?
	Do you have swelling around or below your nipples?	Una uvimbe chuchu chini ya?
	Have you reached change of life?	Je wewe katika wanakuwa wamemaliza?
	Are you having vaginal bleeding?	Unatoka damu ya uke?
	How long have you had the bleeding?	Umetoka damu ya uke kwa muda gani?
	Is the vaginal bleeding continuous or does it come and go?	Unatoka damu ya uke mfululizo au kunakuja na kwenda?
	Have you missed your menstrual period recently?	Umekosa hedhi hivi karibuni?
	Are you pregnant?	Ni mjamzito? (Una mimba?)
	How many months pregnant are you?	Umekuwa mjamzito kwa miezi mingapi?
	Could you possibly be pregnant?	Je, unaweza uwezekano kuwa mjamzito? (Unaweza kuwa na mimba?)
	Can we do a pregnancy test?	Tfanye upimaji wa ujauzito?
	Are your periods regular?	Uko mu wakati ya kupata damu?
	Are your periods painful?	Wakait ya kupata damu unasikia maumivu?
	Is the flow heavy?	Unapata damu mingi?
	When did your last period start?	Uliingia mwezini tarehe gani hivi karibuni? (Hedhi yako mwisho ilikuwa lini?)
	How many days do your periods last?	Siku ngapi kufanya vipindi hedhi ya mwisho?
	Do you bleed between periods?	Je, una damu ya ziada kati ya vipindi hedhi?
	Do you take birth control pills?	Unatumia vidonge vya kuzuia mimba?

Review of systems: Women's Health	English	Swahili
	Do you have an intrauterine device (IUD)?	Una kifaa cha kuzuia mimba?
	Do you have pain during intercourse?	Una maumivu wakati wa kujamiiana?
	Do you have vaginal itching?	Je, una kuwasha uke?
	Do you have vaginal pain?	Uko na uke maumivu?
	Do you have unusual discharge from the vagina; a little or a lot?	Una utoko wowote; kidogo wal mingi?
	How many times have you been pregnant?	Umekuwa na mimba mingapi?
	How many children do you have?	Una watoto wangapi?
	Were your deliveries normal?	Je, alikuwa na ugumu wowote na kujifungua katika siku za nyuma?
	Have you had any miscarriages?	Wewe alikuwa haribikiwa na mimba?
	Did you have problems in your previous pregnancies?	Je, una matatizo yoyote na mimba kabla yako?
	Did you have any severe bleeding after any of your deliveries?	Je, una kutokwa na damu nyingi baada ya kujifungua yako ya mwisho.
	Do you know your blood type?	Damu lako iko kua kikundi gani?
	Do you have ankle swelling?	Je, una uvimbe wa vifundoni?
	Are you in labor?	Una fanya kazi?
	When did your contractions start?	Ulianza kazi lako lini?
	Are the contractions regular or irregular?	Ni uchungu wa kuzaa yako ya si kawaida au kawaida?
	Did your water break?	Ulipoteza maji? (Vunja chupa?)
	Is this your first baby?	Huu ni mtoto wako wa kwanza?
	Do you feel the baby move?	Unasikia mtoto akitembea?
	Do not push.	Usisukume bado.
	Push now.	Sukuma sasa.
	Push very hard.	Sukuma sasa kwa nguvu kadiri uwezavyo.
	You have a boy!	Ni mvulana!
	You have a girl!	Ni msichana!
	You have twins!	Ni mapacha!

Review of systems: Women's Health	English	Swahili
	The baby/babies is/are healthy.	Mtoto/vitoto anaonekana mwenye afya.

Review of systems: neonatal/peripartum

Review of systems: neonatal and peripartum	English	Swahili
	How old is your baby?	Umri gani ni mtoto?
	What was your baby's birth weight?	Mtoto ulizaliure na kilo ngapi?
	How are you feeding the baby, with breast or bottle?	Jinsi wewe kulisha mtoto: kunyonyesha au chupa-kulisha?
	Is the baby nursing well?	Mtoto ananyonya uzuu?
	Has the baby had a convulsion?	Nyu nutoto arizimiya?
	What color was the amniotic fluid?	Maji yaliyo ndani ya rangi gani?
	Were you ill before the delivery?	Walikuwa wewe mgonjwa kabla ya uzazi?
	What is the baby's temperature.	Je, ni joto ya mtoto huyu?
	Your baby is sick.	Mtoto wako ni mgonjwa.
	We need to help your baby.	Tunahitaji kumtunza mtoto wako.
	You can stay with the baby.	Unaweza kukaa na mtoto wako.
	We need to warm the baby up.	Tunahitaji kuongeza mwili wa mtoto joto.
	We need to put the baby under a special light to because the skin color is yellow.	Ni lazima kuweka hii mtoto chini ya mwanga maalum kwa sababu ya ngozi yake ni ya njano.
	We need to give the baby oxygen.	Lazima kutoa mtoto wako oksijeni.
	Does the child cry often?	Haina mtoto kulia sana?
	Is the child gaining weight?	Ni mtoto kupata uzito?
	Does the child have a good appetite?	Haina mtoto kuwa na hamu nzuri?
	Did the child eat today...yesterday?	Mtoto wako alikula leo... jana?
	What kinds of pain does the child complain of?	Mtoto analalamika ya maumivu katika kile mahali?
	Is the child drinking ok?	Ni mtoto wako kunywa bila shida?
	Is the child eating ok?	Je, mtoto wako kula mengi ya chakula?

Review of systems: neonatal and peripartum	English	Swahili
	Have you seen worms in the vomit or stool? (Does he have worms?)	Yeye ana minyoo?
	Did your child pass urine today?	Mtoto wako amekojoa leo?
	Did you child have a stool today/yesterday?	Mtoto wako amekwenda choo leo/ alikwenda choo jana?
	Does he/she have diarrhea?	Mtoto wako amekuwa na ugonjwa wowote wa kuhara?
	Has he/she been vomiting?	Mtoto wako amekuwa akitapika?

Review of systems: neuro & psychiatric

Review of systems: neuro & psychiatric	English	Swahili
	Do you have facial weakness?	Unaregeya ku macho?
	Do you have facial numbness?	Una ganzi yako macho?
	Do you have leg weakness?	Je udhaifu wako mguu?
	Do you have leg numbness?	Una ganzi wako mguu?
	Do you have arm weakness?	Je udhaifu yako ya mkono?
	Do you have arm numbness?	Una ganzi yako ya mkono?
	Did you lose consciousness?	Ulipoteza fahamu?
	Have you had any convulsions?	Umekuwa tetemeko?
	Do you have tremors?	Umekuwa mitikisiko?
	Do you have headaches?	Unapata maumivu ya kichwa?
	Have you had vision loss in one eye?	Je, una upungufu wa kuona katika jicho mmoja tu?
	Do you have problems with your balance?	Je, wanakabiliwa na gumbizi?
	Do you feel dizzy?	Unaona kizunguzungu?
	Do you have problems walking?	Una shida ya kutembea?
	Do you have pain that travels from your buttock down the back of your leg?	Je, una maumivu kwamba safari kutoka kitako yako chini nyuma ya mguu wako?
	Do you have memory problems?	Je, una kumbukumbu maskini?
	Do you have anxiety?	Je, una wasiwasi?
	Do you have depression?	Je, una huzuni?
	How is your mood?	Ni jinsi gani hisia zako?
	Do you hear voices (that others don't hear)?	Una sauti ndani ya kichwa chako?
	Do you sleep well?	Gani unaweza kulala vizuri?

Commands used during the physical exam

English	Swahili
Lay down.	Lala chini.
Sit up (if they are laying down).	Kukaa sawasawa.
Stand up.	Simama.
Sit down.	Kaa chini.
Sit here.	Kukaa chini, hapa.
Open your mouth.	Fumbua mdomo wako.
Show your tongue.	Nionyesheni ulimi wako.
Say "ahh".	Kusema ahh!
Breathe deeply.	Pumua kwa undani.
Close your eyes.	Fumba macho yako.
Raise your eyebrows.	Kuongeza nyushi yako.
Smile widely.	Tabasamu sana.
Swallow now.	Kumeza sasa.
Open your eyes.	Fungua macho yako.
Say "yes" if you feel this.	Unahisi hii? Kusema ndio kama wewe kuhi:
Do this movement (quickly).	Kufanya hili tendo, haraka.
Move your arm like I do.	Hoja mkono wako kama hii.
Lay on your side.	Uongo upande wako.
Lay on your abdomen.	Lala kifudifudi.
Bend your knee.	Pinda goti wako.

Physical exam

Physical exam	English	Swahili
General	Appearance, height	tokeo, kimu cha mtu
Weight	weight (pounds/kilograms) "Stand on the scale."	uzani "Simama juu ya mizani."
Vital signs	pulse, blood pressure "I need to check your blood pressure" respiratory rate	kipigo cha msipa wa damu, msukumo wa damu "Nahitaji kuchukua hali ya shinikizo la dawa lako." kupumua kiwango cha
Vital signs	temperature "Hold this under your tongue."	moto "Shika hiki chini ya ulimi wako."
Skin	skin	ngozi
HEENT	visual acuity "Cover your right eye. Read this. Now, cover your left eye." (Show them a Snellen chart)	Nginsi ya Kuona: "Funika jicho lako la kulia (kuume). Soma hii. Sasa, funika jicho lako la kushoto" (waoneshe chati ya Snellen)
HEENT	conjunctivae, sclerae	ngozi nyembamba inayofunika sehemu ya nje ya jicho ndani ya kope, nyeupe sehemu ya jicho
HEENT	pupils "I am going to shine a light into your eyes."	kiini cha jicho "Nitaangalia machoni mwako ni hii."
HEENT	PERRL pupils equal, round and reactive to light	wakati mboniza macho zimetoshana, ni za mviringo na macho yanaangalia nuru ipasavyo
HEENT	"I am going to put some drops in your eyes."	"Nitaweka dawa ya matone machoni mwako."
HEENT	"You are going to feel a puff of air in your eyes."	"Nitatoa pumzi ya hewa jichoni mwako."
HEENT	optic disc (exam using an ophthalmoscope)	uchunguzi kwa kutumia ophthalmoscope
HEENT	ear canal, tympanic membrane "I am going to look into your ears."	nje ya sikio mfereji. "Mimi ni lazima kuangalia katika masikio yako."
HEENT	AC> BC bilaterally? Rinne. "Cover this ear with your hand. Tell me when you cannot feel the vibration." Move the tuning fork off the mastoid process and next to but not touching the ear. "Tell me when the sound stops."	Rinne mtihani. "Funika sikio hii na mkono wako. Niambie (ni elezee) wakati hauwezi kusikia mtetemeko" "Niambie wakati sauti inaisha"
HEENT	Weber "Is the sound the same in both ears?	Weber mtihani. "Ni sauti moja masikioni?"

Physical exam	English	Swahili
HEENT	nasal mucosa (inside of the nose) "I am going to look into your nose."	(Ndani ya pua) "Mimi ni lazima kuangalia ndani ya pua yako."
HEENT	nasal septum	vya tenganisho la pua
HEENT	soft palate	kaakaa laini
HEENT	sinuses (cavity behind the forehead)	pango au tundu nyuma kipaji
HEENT	teeth	meno
HEENT	1) mouth or lips, 2) gums, 3) teeth, 4)uvula, Stenson's and Wharton's ducts "Open your mouth, please."	1) kinywa au mdomo 2) ufizi 3) meno 4) kimio"Fumbua mdomo wako."
HEENT	"Stick out your tongue please."	"Nionyesheni ulimi wako."
HEENT	"Say ahh!"	"Kusema ahh!"
Chest	Auscultation,(listen to the lungs) "Breathe in deeply."	Sikiliza sauti ya mapafu "Pumua kwa undani."
Chest	percussion "I must tap on your chest- this won't hurt."	"Mimi ni lazima bomba kwenye kifua yako- hii si kuumiza."
Chest	"Lie down on your back, please."	"Lala chali, tafadhali."
Chest	"Lie on your left side."	"Lala kwa upande wa kushoto."
Chest	"Lie on your right side."	"Lala kwa upande wa kulia."
Chest	"Does it hurt here?"	"Je, hii kuumiza?"
Chest	cva tenderness (where the last rib meets the spine)	ambapo ubavu mwisho hukutana mgongo huruma
Chest	heart rate, rhythm "I need to listen to your chest. Breathe normally."	kiwango cha moyo, mahadhi "Mimi ni lazima kusikiliza kifua chako. Kupumua kawaida"
Chest	heart murmur?	moyo msinung'unike
Chest	carotid "Hold your breath."	"Zuia pumzi yako."
Chest	jugular venous pressure (pressure in the neck vein)	shinikizo katika mshipa shingoni mwake
Chest	nipple discharge?	kinyaa cha chuchu
Chest	breast tenderness?	matiti huruma
Chest	breast exam	matiti uchunguzi
Vascular	carotid, radial, aortic pulsation "Hold your breath."	"Zuia pumzi yako."
Vascular	femoral, dorsalis pedis and posterior tibial pulsation (pulsation of legs)	mpapatiko wa miguu
Extremities	leg edema?	uvimbe cha miguu
Extremities	"Lie down please."	"Lala chini, tafadhali."

Physical exam	English	Swahili
Pain	"Show me where it hurts, by touching the spot with one finger."	"Kutumia kidole moja kwa kugusa soa kwamba machungu."
Pain	"Does this hurt?"	"Hii inauma?"
Abdomen	umbilicus	kitovu
Abdomen	inguinal hernia?	kinena ngiri
Abdomen	palpation "I must press my hands on your abdomen."	"Ni lazima ku papasa tumbo yako na mikono yangu."
Abdomen	auscultation "I must listen to your abdomen."	"Nilazima nisikilize sauti ya tumbo."
Abdomen	fluid wave, superficial abdominal veins?	juu juu ya tumbo mishipa
Women's health	Uterine height (cm)	urefu wa mji wa mimba
Women's health	fetal heart tones	moyo tani ya kitoto
Women's health	urinalysis	maabara ya mtihani wa mkojo
Women's health	presentation:	sehemu ya mtoto inayotangulia kutoka wakati wa kuzaliwa
Women's health	face presentation	uso ni inavyoonekana kwanza
Women's health	breech presentation	matako ni umeonyesha kwanza
Women's health	speculum exam	uchungu na speculum
Women's health	vaginal exam	uchunguzi uke
Women's health	gestational age	ujauzito umri
Women's health	amniotic fluid (waters within)	Maji yaliyo ndani
Neonatal	Apgar, 1 minute	alama ya apga
Neonatal	Breathing effort: If the infant is not breathing-score is 0. If the respirations are slow or irregular-score is 1. If the infant cries well-score is 2.	kupumua juhudi: Kama watoto wachanga si kinga-bao ni 0. Kama Kupumua ni mwepesi ni 1. Kama watoto wachanga analia vizuri alama ni 2.
Neonatal	Heart rate evaluated by stethoscope. If there is no heartbeat-score is 0. If the heart rate is less than 100 beats per minute-score is 1. If the heart rate is over 100 beats per minute-score is 2.	kiwango cha moyo kwa kusikiliza moyo. Kama hakuna mapigo ya moyo-bao ni 0. Kama kiwango cha moyo ni chini ya 100 beats kwa dakika alama-ni 1. Kama kiwango cha moyo ni zaidi ya 100 beats kwa dakika alama-ni 2.
Neonatal	Muscle tone. If the muscles are loose and floppy-score is 0. If there is some tone-score is 1. If there is active motion-score is 2.	uimara wa mwili: Kama misuli ni huru na teketeke-bao ni 0. Kama kuna baadhi ya sauti: bao ni 1. Kama kuna kazi mwendo-alama ni 2.

Physical exam	English	Swahili
Neonatal	Grimace response or reflex irritability in response to a mild pinch. If there is no reaction-score is 0. If there is grimacing-score is 1. If there is grimacing and a cough, sneeze, or vigorous cry-score is 2.	usoni ndita baada bana kali. Kama hakuna majibu-bao ni 0. Kama kuna kukunja uso - bao ni 1. Kama kuna kukunja uso na kukohoa, kupiga chafya, au kisayansi kilio-bao ni 2.
Neonatal	Skin color: If the color is pale blue-score is 0. If the body is pink and the extremities blue-score 1. If the entire body is pink-score is 2.	rangi ya ngozi. Kama rangi ni rangi ya bluu-bao ni 0. Kama mwili ni nyekundu na bluu-yamefika bao 1. Kama mwili mzima ni nyekundu-bao ni 2.
Neonatal	Apgar at 5minutes	alama katika dakika 5
Neonatal	Fontanelle	utosi
GU	circumcision?	kutahiri
GU	genital herpes?	malengelenge sehemu za siri
GU	testicular exam	pumbu mtihani
Rectal	hemorrhoids,nodules, prostate on rectal exam	bawasiri, vinundu, tezi kibofu
Rectal	"I want to check your rectum for hemorrhoids. This might be uncomfortable. Bend over please."	"Mimi lazima kuangalia puru yako. Hii inaweza kuwa na wasiwasi. Konda kwenye meza tafadhali."
Rectal	guaiac:positive or negative	mtihani kwa ajili ya damu katika kinyesi: chanya au hasi
Neurology	"Sit up please."	"Kukaa sawasawa, tafadhali."
Neurology	N1 Olfactory: coffee, peppermint? "Close your eyes and tell me what you smell."	kahawa, peremende?"Fumba macho yako...nini wewe harufu?"
Neurology	N2 Optic: Snellen chart confrontation. "Read the letters on this chart. Follow my finger with your eyes, without moving your head."	"Kusoma hii. Kufuata kidole yangu na macho yako, bila ya kusonga kichwa yako."
Neurology	N3,4,6 Oculomotor, Trochlear, Abducens. EOM's "Follow my finger."	"Angalia kidole changu kinaposonga."
Neurology	N5 Trigeminal "Clench your jaw." "Move your jaw back and forth."	"Karibu mdomo wako kukazwa." "Hoja ya taya yako upande kwa upande."
Neurology	Ophthalmic branch: forehead, Maxillary branch: cheek, Mandibular branch: chin, "Do you feel this?"	paji la uso, shavu, kidevu "Unahisi hii?"

Physical exam	English	Swahili
Neurology	N7 Facial: "Raise your eyebrows."	"Kuongeza nyushi yako."
Neurology	"Close your eyes tightly, smile big."	"Karibu na macho yako kukazwa, tabasamu sana."
Neurology	N8 Acoustic: whisper, Rinne "Can you hear me talking? Try to repeat what I say."	"Unaweza kusikia mimi kuzungumza? Kurudia kile alisema."
Neurology	"Tell me when you can't feel the vibration."	"Niambie wakati huwezi kuhisi mteteko."
Neurology	N9 Glossopharyngeal: swallow (hoarseness?) "Swallow please."	"Kumeza sasa, tafadhali."
Neurology	N10 Vagus: swallow, soft palate, gag reflex "Open your mouth widely. Stick out your tongue please. Now, close it."	"Kufungua mdomo wako. Nionyesheni ulimi wako. Sasa, karibu mdomo wako."
Neurology	N11 Spinal accessory nerve: "Turn your head to the right, now to the left. Shrug your shoulders.(like this)"	"Kugeuza kichwa yako ya haki. Sasa, kurejea kichwa yako ya kushoto. Kuongeza mabega yako. (kama hii)"
Neurology	N12 Hypoglossal: tongue midline	ulimi ni katikati
Neurology	Glasgow coma score	Glasgow kukosa fahamu wadogo
Neurology	Opens eyes to: spontaneous (4), to speech (3), to pain (2), none (1)	jicho ufunguzi: hiari (4), katika kukabiliana na hotuba (3), kitika kukabiliana na maumivu (2), hakuna (1)
Neurology	Best motor: "Hold up two fingers" obeys commands (6), localizes:reaches for the part of the body being stimulated (5), withdraws (4), abnormal flexion (3), abnormal extension (2), none (1)	misuli majibu: "Nionyesheni vidole viwili." kumt'ii amri (6), fika kuelekea eneo hilo kunasababishwa (5), hujiondoa kutoka eneo kunasababishwa (4), hali isiyo ya kawaida kunyumbua mkono (3), hali isiyo ya kawaida kupanua mkono (2), hakuna (1)
Neurology	Best verbal: oriented (5), confused (4), inappropriate (3), garbled (2), none (1)	matusi majibu: kiakili husika (5), kuchanganyikiwa (4), lisilohusiana na mada ya mjadala (3), kuumbuka (2), hakuna (1)
Neurology	Motor function	misuli kazi
Neurology	biceps brachii, elbow flexion "Pull your arm up, like this."	"Pinda mkono wako, kama hii."
Neurology	wrist extensors "Bend your wrist up, like this."	"Pinda kiwiko cha mkono wako, kama hii."

Physical exam	English	Swahili
Neurology	triceps brachii, elbow extension "Straighten your arm out, like this."	"Nyorosha mkono wako, kama hii."
Neurology	finger flexors, distal phalanx middle finger "bend the tip of this finger"	"Pinda ncha ya kidole hii."
Neurology	finger abduction, little finger "hold the small finger tightly. (Don't let me squeeze your fingers together.)"	"Kuenea vidole. Wala naomba itapunguza vidole pamoja."
Neurology	iliopsoas, hip flexors "Move this knee to your chest, now the other knee."	"Hoja ya goti lako na kifua chako. Sasa kurudia na goti nyingine."
Neurology	quadriceps, knee extensors "Straighten your leg out, like this."	"Nyorosha mguu lako. Sasa kurudia na mguu nyingine."
Neurology	tibialis anterior, ankle dorsiflexors "Pull your foot up, like this."	"Kuvuta au pandisha mguu wako juu, kama hii."
Neurology	extensor hallucis longus, long toe extension "Raise your toe up, like this."	"Kuvuta au pandisha gumba lako, kama hii."
Neurology	gastrocnemius, ankle plantar flexors "Push your foot down against my hand, like this."	"Kushinikiza chini ya mguu yako dhidi ya mkono wangu,kama hii"
Neurology	"Is the sensation dull or sharp? Say sharp or dull."	"Je, hii kujisikia makali au wepesi?
Neurology	C-4 (top of acromioclavicular joint)	(juu ya bega pamoja)
Neurology	C-5 (lateral side of antecubital fossa)	(imara nyanja ya kiwiko)
Neurology	C-6 (thumb)	(gumba)
Neurology	C-7 (middle finger)	(tatu kidole)
Neurology	C-8 (little finger)	(tano kidole)
Neurology	T-4 (nipple line)	(katika ngazi ya chuchu)
Neurology	T-10 (umbilicus)	(kitovu)
Neurology	L-2 (mid-anterior thigh)	(mbele na katikati sehemu ya paja)
Neurology	L-3 (medial femoral condyle)	(sehemu ya goti ijayo karibu na goti nyingine)
Neurology	L-4 (medial malleolus)	(sehemu ya kifundo cha mguu ijayo karibu na kifundo cha mguu nyingine)
Neurology	L-5 (dorsum of the foot, at third MTP joint)	(juu ya mguu karibu kidole ya tatu cha mguu)
Neurology	S-1 (Lateral heel)	(imara nyanja ya kisigno)

Physical exam	English	Swahili
Neurology	S-2 (popliteal fossa of the knee, in the midline)	(nyuma ya goti katikati)
Neurology	S-3 (ischial tuberosity)	(mfupa umaarufu kwamba mmoja aketiye juu ya)
Neurology	S4-5 (perianal area)	(karibu mkundu)
Neurology	Reflexes; "I am going to tap you here with this reflex hammer."	tendo la mwili lisiloweza kuzuiwa: "Mimi ni lazima upole kugusa wewe kwa nyundo hii " "Ninataka kukupiga (kugonga) kwa upole na hama (nyundo) hii."
Neurology	triceps right and left	karibu kishingo cha mkono: kulia na kushoto
Neurology	biceps, right and left	saa hangue ya mkono; kulia na kushoto
Neurology	brachioradial, right and left	katika kiganja karibu gumba; kulia na kushoto
Neurology	patella, right and left	kilegesambwa; kulia na kushoto
Neurology	ankle, right and left	kifundo cha mguu; kulia na kushoto
Neurology	babinski, right and left (great toe extension= positive)	kulia na kushoto (kidole cha mguu kupanuliwa = usiokuwa wa kawaida)
Neurology	**Tandem walk** "Walk like this, one foot in front of other." (Or, say walk like this and demonstrate.)	"Tembea kama hii."
Neurology	**heel walk, toe walk** "Walk on your heels, now walk on your toes."	"Tembeleya ku visingino ya miguu, tembeleya vidole ya miguu."
Neurology	**romberg** "Stand up, hold your arms out, close your eyes."	"Simama, panua mikono yako, funga macho yako."
Neurology	**rapid alternating movement** (2nd finger, thumb) "Do this, fast".	"Kufanya hili tendo, haraka."
Neurology	**heel-shin** "Close your eyes. Move your right heel from your left knee to the ankle. Now, move your left heel from your right knee down to the ankle." (Open your eyes, let me demonstrate.)	"Fumba macho yako. Hoja ya kulia kisigino kutoka goti wako wa kushoto kwa mguu. (Sasa,kuangalia mimi; kurudia hatua yangu.)
Neurology	**finger nose finger** "Touch my finger with your finger then touch your nose."	"Kugusa kidole changu kidole kisha kugusa pua yako."

Physical exam	English	Swahili
Neurology	**stereognosis** (key, pencil, cup) "Close your eyes; what is this in your hand?"	(ufunguo, kalamu ya risasi, kikombe) "Fumba macho yako: niambie nini kuhisi katika mkono wako."
Neurology	**graphesthesia** (draw #3 in hand) "Close your eyes, what is the number written in your hand?"	"Fumba macho yako. Je, ni idadi niliandika katika mkono wako?"
Neurology	**point localization**: "Close your eyes, tell me what part of your body is being touched."	"Fumba macho yako. Kuniambia nin sehemu ya mwili wako mimi kugusa."
Neurology	**two point discrimination**: "Do you feel one or two points of contact?"	"Je, unajisikia moja sindano au mbili?"
Mental status	SLUMS Examination	SLUMS
Mental status	Saint Louis University Mental Status Examination	Chuo Kikuu cha St Louis uchunguzi ya Hali ya akili.
Mental status	What day of the week is it? (1)	Leo, nisikugani ya wiki? (1) (Ni siku gani ya wiki leo?
Mental status	What is the year? (1)	Ni mwaka gani? (1) Tuko mwaka gani?
Mental status	What state are we in? (1)	Ni katika mji gani sisi tunaishi(tuko)? (1) Tunaikala mu muji gani?
Mental status	Please remember these five objects. I will ask you what they are later. Pineapple Pen Hat House Car	Tafadhali, kumbuka izi vitu tano. Nitawauliza vitu hii baadaye: nanasi, kalamu kofia, nyumba, gari
Mental status	You have 1000 Congolese francs and you go to the store and buy a dozen mangoes for 300 francs and fabric for 200francs. How much did you spend? (1) How much do you have left? (2)	Uko na 1000 (helfu moja) ya faranga ya Congo, unaenda ku duka. Una nunua hembe 12 (kumi nambili) ku beyi ya 300 (miya tatu), unauza kitambaa ya 200 (miya mbili). Ulitumikisha (ulitumia) pesa ngapi? (1) Unabakiya (unabaki) na pesa ngapi?(2)
Mental status	Please name as many animals as you can in one minute. (0) 0-4 animals, (1) 5-9 animals, (2) 10-14 animals, (3) 15+ animals	Tafadhali, ni jina ngapi ya wanyama unaweza taja mu dakika moja. (0) wanyama0-4, (1) wanyama 5-9, (2) wanyama 10-14, (3) wanyama 15+
Mental status	What were the five objects I asked you to remember? pineapple Pen Tie House Car. One point for each correct answer.	Ni vitu tano gani nili kuambia unikumbushe? nanasi, kalamu, kofia, nyumba, gari. Alama moja kukila jibu la kweli.

Physical exam	English	Swahili
Mental status	I am going to give you a series of numbers and I would like you to give them to me backwards. For example, if I say 42, you say 24. (0) 87, (1) 649, (2) 8537	Ninaenda kusema mfululizo wa namba; Ningependa unipe tena iyo mfululizo wa namba kuanza nyuma una rudi mbele. Kwa mfano, kama na sema 24, una sema 42. (0) 87, (1) 649, (2) 8537
Mental status	This is a clock face. Please put in the hour markers and the time at ten minutes to eleven o'clock. (2) Hour markers correct? (2) Time correct?	Hii ni picha ya saa. Tafadhali weka alama za saa katika saa na wakati katika dakika kumi kabla ya 11:00 (saa tano). (2) Alama ya saa ni sahihi?. (2) Muda ni sahihi.
Mental status	Place an X in the triangle. □△◇, (1) Which of the figures is the largest? (1)	Weka alama juu ya pembetatu. (1)Takwimu kubwa ni gapi? (1)
Mental status	I am going to read you a story. Please listen carefully because afterwards, I'm going to ask you some questions about it. Jill was a very successful doctor. She made a lot of money on the stock market. She then met Jack, a strong man. She married him and had three children. They lived in Goma. She then stopped work and stayed at home to bring up her children. When they were teenagers, she went back to work. She and Jack lived happily ever after.	Nataka kuwasomea hadisi. Tafazali, sikilizeni kwa makini kwa sababu baadae nita wauliza maswali kuhusu hilo. Jill alikuwa daktari (munganga) wa mafanikio sana. Amepata pesa nyingi kwenyi soko. Kisha alikutana na Jack, mwanaume myenye nguvu. Akaolewa naye na akapata wototo watatu. Wailishi (katika mji wa) Goma. Kisha akaacha kazi, akabaki nyumbani kuwa komalisha watoto. Wakati hawa watoto walikuwa na myaka kumi na zaidi, akarudi kutumika. Yeye na Jack wakaishi maisha ya heri siku zote baadaye.
Mental status	What was the female's name? (2)	Jina la msichana (binti) ni gani? (2)
Mental status	What work did she do? (2)	Ni kazi gani alikuwa (Jill) na tumika? (2)
Mental status	When did she go back to work? (2)	Wakati gani alirudi(Jill) kufanya kazi? (2)
Mental status	What state did she live in? (2)	Katika mji gani alikuwa (Jill) anaishi? (2)
Mental status	Add total score, with high school education: 27-30 normal, 21-26 mild cognitive disorder, 1-20 dementia. Without high school education: 25-30 normal, 20-24 mild cognitive disorder, 1-19 dementia.	alama ya jumla, na elimu ya shule ya sekondari: 27-30 kawaida, 21-26 kali utambuzi machafuko, 1-20 shida ya akili. Bila elimu ya shule ya sekondari: 25-30 kawaida, 20-24 kali utambuzi machafuko, 1-19 shida ya akili.

Joint exam

Joint exam	English	Swahili
	Shoulder test for impingement. Apley scratch test: Use your right hand to touch the left scapula by reaching over the left clavicle. Next, use your right hand to touch the right scapula. Thirdly, move your right thumb to the middle of your back between the scapulae. **"Move your arm like I do"**	**"Hoja mkono wako kama hii."**
	Shoulder test for impingement.Neers test: Place one hand on the patient's scapula, grasp their forearm with your other hand (their thumb should be facing down). Slowly forward flex the arm. **"I am going to put my hand on your shoulder blade and move your arm."**	**"Mimi lazima kugusa bega wako au hoja mkono wako."**
	Supraspinatus isometric test: the patient holds their arm at 20 degrees abduction and the examiner attempts adduction. **"Hold your arm like this and try to raise it."**	**"Kushikilia mkono wako kama hii. Sana, kuinua mkono wako."**
	Supraspinatus function. Painful arc sign: **"I am going to raise your arm, let me know when you have pain."**	**"Mimi lazima kuinua mkono wako. Una mauvimo?"**
	Supraspinatus function. Drop arm test: raise the arm to 180 degrees abduction then instruct the patient: **"Slowly lower your arm to your side".** If the arm falls quickly the test is positive.	**"Pole pole, kuacha mkono wako."**
	Supraspinatus function. Jobe's or empty can test: hold the arm straight at the elbow at 90 degrees abduction, 30 degrees forward flexion and internally rotate the shoulder. Hand the patient a cup and instruct: **"Turn this cup upside down."** Pain during this motion is a positive sign.	**"Kugeuka kikombe hiki kichwa chini."**
	External rotation test for infraspinatus impingement. Have the patient abduct the shoulders 30 degrees, flex at the elbow 90 degrees. Hold the outside of the forearm and direct them to **"Push outward.(against me)"**	**"Jisukume kwanga."**

Joint exam	English	Swahili
	Subscapularis;Push off test: have the patient put their arm behind their back with the palm facing outward and push against the examiner's hand. **"Move your hand like this and push against my hand."**	**"Hoja kofi wako kama hii, na jisukume kwanga."**
	Tinel test for ulnar nerve entrapment: tap over the ulnar groove and ask **"Do you have pain or numbness. If so, where?"** (Pain and numbness at 4th, 5th fingers indicates a positive test.)	**"Una maumivu au ganzi; wapi?"**
	Phalen maneuver for carpal tunnel syndrome: hold the wrist in forced flexion. Pain is a positive indication. **"Do you have pain, where?"**	**"Una maumivu au ganzi; wapi?"**
	Finkelstein test for de Quervain's tenosynovitis. Have the patient cover the thumb with their fingers of the same hand. Deviate the wrist towards the ulna. Pain is indicative of tenosynovitis. **"Hold your hand like this. Does this hurt?"**	**"Kushikilia kofi wako kama hii. Unasikia maumivu ninapofanya hivi?"**
	Scaphoid compression test. The thumb is held and pushed toward the scaphoid. Pain indicates a possible scaphoid fracture. **"Do you feel pain."**	**"Una maumivu?"**
	Hip assessment. Perform internal and external rotation of the hip and ask, **"Does this hurt?"**	**"Unasikia maumivu ninapofanya hivi?"**
	Patrick test for hip or sacroiliac pathology: examiner flexes, abducts, externally rotates and extends the leg so that the ankle of that leg is on top of the opposite knee. **"I am going to move your leg, does this hurt?"**	**"Mimi lazima hoja mguu wako; una maumiva."**
	Piriformis test Patient is in lateral decubitus position with hip flexed at 60 degrees and knee at full extension. Examiner places a hand on the patient's shoulder and exerts mild pressure on the flexed leg at the knee. A positive test is noted by radicular pain caused by impingement of the sciatic nerve by the tight piriformis muscle. **"Lay on your left side, and now, lay on your right side."**	**"Lala kua upande wa kushoto, na sasa, lala kua upande wa kulia."**

Joint exam	English	Swahili
	Ely's test to assess rectus femoris flexibility. Patient lays prone with legs fully extended. Examiner passively flexes the knee to full ROM. If the ipsilateral hip rises it is suggestive of a tight rectus femoris muscle. **"Lay on your abdomen."**	**"Lala kifudifudi."**
	Fulcrum test Patient is seated on a table with legs dangling. Examiner places their forearm under the thigh for use as a fulcrum. Pressure is applied with the other hand over the knee and up the femur. Pain elicited may indicate a stress fracture. **"Sit on the edge of the bed."**	**"Kukaa juu ya upande wa kitanda."**
	Straight leg raise **"Lay down, I am going to lift your leg, let me know where you feel pain."**	**"Lala bilakupinda, mimi lazima kuniua mguu wako. Wapi kuhisi maumivo?"**
	Sensation of anterolateral thigh to assess for meralgia paresthetica; **"I am going to touch you with this cotton ball. Do you feel it?"**	**"Mimi lazima kugusa ngozi yako na mpira hii pamba. Unahisi yake?"**
	Knee collateral ligament assessment. valgus stress for medial instability. **"Lay down. I am going to check your knee."** Place one hand on lateral thigh while the other hand is used to apply outward pressure on the calf.	**"Lala chali, mimi lazima kuchunguza goti lako."**
	Knee collateral ligament assessment. varus stress for lateral instability **"Lay down. I am going to check your knee."** Place one hand on the medial thigh while the other hand is used to apply inward pressure on the calf.	**"Lala chali, mimi lazima kuchunguza goti lako."**
	Lachman's test for anterior cruciate ligament injury (ACL) **"Lay down, bend your knee."** Place the knee at 30 degrees flexion, stabilize the the femur with one hand while pulling the proximal tibia anteriorly. Laxity indicates ACL injury.	**"Lala chali, pinda goti wako."**
	Pivot shift test for ACL injury. **"Lay down."** With the knee in full extension the examiner rotates the tibia and applies valgus stress then flexes the knee. If acl injury is present a "clunk" sound will be heard.	**"Lala chali."**

Joint exam	English	Swahili
	Anterior drawer for ACL injury. **"Lay down and bend your knee."** to 90 degrees. The examiner hold the proximal tibia with both hands, sits on the patient's foot and pulls the tibia anteriorly to look for laxity.	**"Lala chali, pinda goti wako."**
	Posterior drawer test for posterior cruciate ligament injury (PCL) Patient is supine with the hips flexed at 45 degrees and knees at 90 degrees, Examiner sits on the patient's feet, grasps the tibia with both hands and applies backward pressure. Laxity is a sign of a torn posterior cruciate ligament. **"Lay on your back and bend your knee."**	**"Lala chali, pinda goti wako."**
	Thessaly test: for knee meniscal injury**"Stand up. Bend your knee and then turn it like this."** Patient should hold the examiner's hand, stand on one leg with the knee flexed at 20 degrees. The patient then internally and externally rotates their knees. Pain or locking is a positive test.	**"Simama, pinda goti wako kama hii."**
	Apley test for knee meniscal injury **"Lay on your abdomen."** With patient prone bend the knee to 90 degrees and apply downward pressure while internally and externally rotating the foot. Pain indicates a positive test.	**"Lala kifudifudi."**
	Ottawa knee rules X ray indicated if any of following are present: 1. age over 55 "What is your age?" 2. Tenderness of patella: "Do you have pain here?" 3. Tenderness of fibular head: "Do you have pain here." Inability to flex the knee to 90 degrees: "4. Bend your knee as much as possible." 5. Inability to transfer weight to each leg. "Stand on your right leg only, now on your left leg only."	1. Unaumri gani? 2. Una maumivu goti? 3. Una maumivu hapi? 4. Pina goti wako sana! 5. Kusimama juu ya mguu wako wa kulia. Na sana, kusimama juu ya mguu wako wa kushoto.
	Ottawa ankle rules, part 1. An ankle x ray is indicated if there is inability to bear weight in the ER or there is tenderness at the posterior edge or tip of the medial or lateral malleolus (distal 6cm). **"Can you walk? Do you have pain when I touch here?"**	**"Unaweza kutembea? Una maumiva hapi?"**

41

Joint exam	English	Swahili
	Ottawa ankle rules, part 2. A foot x ray is indicated if there is inability to bear weight in the ER or there is tenderness at the base of the 5th metatarsal or over the navicular bone. **"Can you walk? Do you have pain when I touch here?"**	**"Unaweza kutembea? Una maumiva hapi?"**
	Thompson test for achilles tendon rupture. The patient lays prone with their feet hanging over the end of the bed. The calf muscles are squeezed and if the Achilles tendon is ruptured there is no plantar flexion of the foot.**"Lay on your abdomen."**	**"Lala kifudifudi."**

Counseling

Counseling	English	Swahili
Pulmonary	You need to go for an x ray.	Unahitaji eksirei ya kifua chako.
	I have the result of your sputum.	Nina matokeo ya mtihani makohozi yako.
	You have...	Una...
	tuberculosis	kifua kikuu
	pneumonia	kamata
	Your lungs are affected, you need to quit smoking today.	Mapafu yako ni walioathirika, unahitaji kuacha sigara leo.
	You must stop smoking.	Lazima usivute sigara.
Infectious disease	You are sick with malaria.	Wewe ni mateso kutokana na malaria.
	You have typhoid fever.	Wewe ni mateso kutokana homa ya matumbo.
	You have intestinal worms.	Wewe ni mateso kutokana na minyoo.
	It will take time for you to heal.	Utahitaji muda kupona.
Gastroenterology	There is an ulcer in your stomach.	Kuna kidonda katika tumbo yako.
	You need to quit drinking beer completely.	Lazima si kunywa pombe, kabisi!
	You have a tumor in your stomach.	Una kansa katika tumbo yako.
	I need to put a suppository in your rectum.	Lazima nitie kidonge katika haja kubua yako.
Surgery	We need to take you to surgery.	Tunahitaji kukupeleka kwenye upasuaji.
	When have you last eaten?	Ulikula chakula chako cha mwisho lini?
	Have you eaten in the last six hours?	Umekula chakula mnamo masaa sita yaliyopita?
	Do not eat or drink until after surgery.	Usile wala kunywa mpaka opereshen.
	I need to have sew up (suture) this wound.	Lazima ya mshono kuziba jeraha. (Nahitaji kukushona mishono kaadha.)
	You are badly injured.	Umeumizwa vibea.
	The operation went very well.	Operesheni ilifanikiwa.
	You need to stay in bed.	Lazima ubaki kitandani.

Counseling	English	Swahili
	You need to stay in the hospital.	Unatakiwa kulala hospitali.
	I need to change your dressing.	Lazami nibadilishe bendeji zako za vidonda.
Pharmacy	I will give you medication.	Nahitaji kukupa dawa.
	This medicine is for pain.	Dawa hii ni ya maumivu.
	This medicine is for the infection.	Dawa hii itapambana na maambukizo.
	Do not drink alcohol while on this medicine.	Epuka pombe wakati unapotumia dawa.
	You take this medicine a) once b) two, c) three, d)four times per day.	Chukua dawa hii a) mara moja kila siku b) mara mbili kila siku c) mara tatu kila siku d) mara nne kila siku
	Take this medicine until the bottle is empty.	Meza hadi imekwisha.
	Take this medication twice a day only if you need to.	Chukua dawa hii mara mbili kila siku kama inavyohitajika.
	Take this medication before eating.	Meza kabla ya kula.
	Take this medication with food.	Meza na chakula.
	Take this medication on an empty stomach.(an hour before or two hours after a meal)	Meza kwa tumbo topu. (saa moja kabla au saa mbili baada ya chakula)
	Take this medicine a) each morning b) each night.	Chukua dawa hii a) kila asubuhi b) kila usiku.
	Take this medicine for a) one week, b) for one (1), two (2), three (3) days.	Chukua dawa hii a) kwa wiki moja b) kwa moja siku (1), mbili siku (2), tatu siku (3) .
	Take this medication after meals.	Mez baada ya kula.
	Take this medication in the morning.	Chukua dawa hii wakati wa asubuhi.
	Take this medication at night.	Chukua dawa hii wakati wa usiku.
	This medicine may change the color of your urine.	Dawa hii inaweza kubadilisha rangi ya kojo au mavi.
	Do not take this with dairy products.	Epuka kutumia wakati mmoja na vyakula vya maziwa.
	Place drops in your bad ear.	Tia matone katika sehemu linalouma.
	Unwrap and insert one suppository in your rectum.	Fungau na uingize kidonge kimoja katika sehemu ya haja kubwa.
	Spray this in your nose.	Nyunyizia katika pua.

Counseling	English	Swahili
	Inhale by mouth (like this).	Vuta pumzi kwa mdomo (kama hii).
	Insert the suppository into your vagina.	Ingiza kidonge kimoja kwa uke.
	Place drops in this eye.	Tia matone katika jicho hii.
	Rub onto your skin.	Paka kwa ngozi.
Maternity/Ob	Congratulations, you are pregnant!	Hongera, una mimba.
	The baby is due on this date...	Mtoto pengine kuwa alizaliwa katika tarehe hii...
	The nurse is on her way.	Mkunga ni juu ya njia yake.
	She will help with the delivery.	Yeye itasaidia na kujifungua.
	You had a boy. You had a girl.	Wewe alikuwa kijana. Wewe alikuwa msichana.
	You had twins.	Wewe alikuwa mapacha.
	You will need a cesarean section.	Utakuwa kuhitaji upasuaji wa kutoa mtoto.
Procedures	"I need to take a blood sample."	Nahitaji kuchukua sampluli ya damu lako kwa uchunguzi.
	"Please give me a urine sample in this cup."	Kojoa ndani ya chombo hiki.
	I need to put a tube in your bladder to drain the urine.	Nitaingiza tyubu katika kobofu chako kuondoa mkojo.
	"Please give me a stool specimen in this container."	Tafadhali nipe sampuli ya kinyesi yako katika kikombe hiki.
	"Please give me a sputum sample in this cup."	"Kohoa kohozi katika kikombe hiki."
	"I need to put this tube in your nose-it will go into your stomach"	"Nahitaji kuweka tyubu kupitia pua yako kwenda tumbo lako."
	"This tube will drain your stomach."	"Tyubu hii itasafisha tumbo yako."
	"You need to swallow to help the tube go in."	"Unahitaji kumeza wakati ninapotia tyubu hii katika pua yako."
	"I need to put a tube in your chest."	"Nahitaki kuweka tyubu ndani ya kibua chako."
	"This tube will drain the air and fluid out of your chest."	"Sindano hii itafungua hewa kutoka kifua chako."
	"I need to start an IV."	"Iazima nikuweke sindano ndogo hapa."
	"We need to give you fluid."	"Tunahitaji kukupatia kitu cha majimaji."
	" We need to give you blood."	"Tunhitaji kukupatia damu."

Counseling	English	Swahili
	I need to give you a shot 1) in the arm, 2) in the leg	Nitadunga sidano mkononi/mguu mwako kikupa dawa.
Orthopedics	You need an x ray of the bone.	Unahitaji ekserei ya mfupa wako.
	You have a broken leg.	Mguu wako ni kuvunjwa.
	You have a broken ankle.	Umevunjika kifundo la mguu.
	You have a broken arm.	Mkono wako ni kuvunjwa.
	You have a broken wrist.	Umevunjika kifundo cha mkono.
	You have fluid in your joint.	Una maji katika pamoja yako. (Una maji katika yako kiungo.)
	You need a cast.	Unahitaji plasta kusaidia mfupa kupona.
	Do not remove or get the cast wet.	Usitoe au usilowe plasta.
	I need to splint your arm/leg.	Nahitaki kufunga mkono/mguu walko kwa banzi.
	You may take the splint off to bathe but it must be put back on afterwards.	Unaweza kutoa banzi ili kujisafisha lakini lazima banzi lirudishwe mahali pake baada ya wewe kujisafisha.
	We need to do surgery to place a metal plate with screws to help the bone heal.	Unahitai chuma na skrubu kasaidia kupona kwa mfupa wako.
Pediatrics	Your child looks fine.	Mtoto wako anaonekana mwenye afya nzuri.
	Your child will be ill for quite a while.	Mtoto wako atakuwa mgonjwa kwa muda mrefu.
	Give the child small amounts of food every few hours.	Mlishe mtoto vipande vidogo kila masaa machache.
	Give your child this to drink every few hours.	Msaidie mtoto wako kunywa hii kila masaa machache.
	It is ok to let your child sleep.	Ruhusu mtoto wako kulala.
	Bring your child back to the clinic tomorrow.	Mrudishe mtoto wako hapa kesho.
General	What you have is not serious.	Wewe si mgonjwa sana.
	You will be better soon.	Utapata nafuu hivi karibuni.
	Don't worry, you'll get better.	Usijali utapona.
	Your condition is grave.	Wewe ni mgonjwa mahutui.
	Please come back if you have more problems.	Rudi mnamo kama una matatizo.
	Please return in one week.	Rudi mnamo wiki moja, tafadhali.

46

Date/time, numbers

Date/time, numbers	English	Swahili
	January	mwezi wa kwanza
	February	mwezi wa pili
	March	mwezi wa tatu
	April	mwezi wa nne
	May	mwezi wa tano
	June	mwezi wa sita
	July	mwezi wa saba
	August	mwezi wa nane
	September	mwezi wa tisa
	October	mwezi wa kumi
	November	mwezi wa kumi na moja
	December	mwezi wa kumi na mbili
	Sunday	jumapili
	Monday	jumatatu
	Tuesday	jumanne
	Wednesday	jumatano
	Thursday	alhamisi
	Friday	ijumaa
	Saturday	jumamosi
	0 (zero)	sifuri
	1 one	moja
	2 two	mbili
	3 three	tatu
	4 four	nne
	5 five	tano
	6 six	sita
	7 seven	saba
	8 eight	nane
	9 nine	tisa
	10 ten	kumi
	11 eleven	kumi na moja
	12 twelve	kumi na mbili
	13 thirteen	kumi na tatu
	14 fourteen	kumi na nne
	15 fifteen	kumi na tano
	16 sixteen	kumi na sita
	17 seventeen	kumi na saba

Date/time, numbers	English	Swahili
	18 eighteen	kumi na nane
	19 nineteen	kumi na tisa
	20 twenty	ishirini
	21 twenty-one	ishirini na moja
	30 thirty	thelathini
	31 thirty-one	thelathini na moja
	40 forty	arobaini
	50 fifty	hamsini
	60 sixty	sitini
	70 seventy	sabini
	71 seventy-one	sabini na moja
	72 seventy-two	sabini na mbili
	73 seventy-three	sabini na tatu
	74 seventy-four	sabini na nne
	75 seventy-five	sabini na tano
	76 seventy-six	sabini na sita
	77 seventy-seven	sabini na saba
	78 seventy-eight	sabini na nane
	79 seventy-nine	sabini na kenda
	80 eighty	themanini
	81 eighty-one	themanini na moja
	82 eighty-two	themanini na mbili
	90 ninety	tisini
	91 ninety-one	tisini na moja
	92 ninety-two	tisini na mbili
	100 one hundred	mia moja
	200 two hundred	mia mbili
	300 three hundred	mia tatu
	400 four hundred	mia nne
	500 five hundred	mia tano
	600 six hundred	mia sita
	700 seven hundred	mia saba
	800 eight hundred	mia nane
	900 nine hundred	mia kenda
	1000 one thousand	elfu moja
	1500 one thousand five hundred	elfu moja mia tano
	2000 two thousand	elfu mbili
	2500 two thousand five hundred	elfu mbili mia tano
	5000 five thousand	elfu tano

Date/time, numbers	English	Swahili
	At what time?	Saa ngapi?
	At 8p.m. (this evening)	Saa mbili usika.
	At noon.	Saa sita mchana.
	It is 9 a.m.	Ni saa tatu asubuhi.
	It is 2:30 p.m.	Ni saa nane na nusu mchana.
	It is 7:15 a.m.	Ni saa moja na robo asubuhi.
	It is 10:45 a.m.	Ni saa tano kasarobo.
	today	leo
	tomorrow	kesho
	yesterday	jana
	soon	karibu
	right now	sasa hivi
	now	sasa
	morning	asubuhi
	noon	adhuhuri
	afternoon	mchana
	evening	jioni
	midnight	saa sita usiku
	night	usiku
	last week	juma jana
	this week	wiki hii
	next week	juma kesho
	last year	mwaka jana
	this year	mwaka huu
	next year	mwaka kesho
	one week	wiki moja
	two weeks	wiki mbili
	one month	mwezi mmoja
	two months	mwezi mbili
	three months	mwezi tatu
	four months	mwezi manne
	five months	mwezi tano

Body parts

Body parts	English	Swahili
HEENT	head	kichwa
HEENT	skull	fuu la kichwa
HEENT	hair	nywele
HEENT	forehead	paji la uso; kipaji
HEENT	face	uso
HEENT	eye (eyes)	jicho (macho)
HEENT	pupil	kiini cha jicho
HEENT	eyebrow (eyebrows)	ushi (nyushi)
HEENT	eyelash/eyelid	ukope
HEENT	nose	pua
HEENT	nostril (nostrils)	tunda la pua (matunda ya mapua)
HEENT	ear (ears)	sikio (masikio)
HEENT	earlobe	ndewe
HEENT	tongue	ulimi
HEENT	tooth (teeth)	jino (meno)
HEENT	cheek	shavu
HEENT	lips	midomo
HEENT	tonsils	kifuko
HEENT	throat	koo
HEENT	mouth	mdomo
HEENT	chin	kidevu
HEENT	mandible	taya
HEENT	neck (anterior)	shingo
HEENT	adam's apple	kikoromeo
Upper limbs	clavicle	mtulinga
Upper limbs	shoulder (shoulders)	bega (mabega)
Upper limbs	axilla	kwapa
Upper limbs	humerus	mfupa wa mkono katikati ya kiko na bega
Upper limbs	arm (arms)	mkono (mikono)
Upper limbs	upper arm	ya juu ya mkono
Upper limbs	elbow (elbows)	kiwiko, kisugudi (visugudi);
Upper limbs	lower arm	kigasha
Upper limbs	wrist	kilimbili
Upper limbs	palm of hand	kiganja
Upper limbs	hand (hands)	mkono; kofi
Upper limbs	thumb	dole gumba au kidole cha gumba
Upper limbs	finger (fingers)	kidole (vidole)

Body parts	English	Swahili
Upper limbs	5th finger	tano kidole au kidole cha mwisho
Upper limbs	4th finger	nne kidole au kidole cha kando
Upper limbs	3rd finger	tatu kidole au kidole cha kati
Upper limbs	2nd finger	pili kidole au kidole cha shadada
Upper limbs	knuckle	nguyu
Upper limbs	fingernail	ukucha wa kidole cha mkono
Thorax	lower back	mgongo
Thorax	scapula	kombe; fuzi
Thorax	chest	kifua
Thorax	rib (ribs)	ubavu (mbavu)
Thorax	heart	moyo
Thorax	lung (lungs)	pafu (mapafu)
Thorax	breast (breasts)	(maziwa)
Thorax	nipple	chuchu; kilembwa cha titi
Abdomen	abdomen	fumbatio
Abdomen	esophagus	umio wa chakula
Abdomen	liver	maini
Abdomen	stomach	tumbo
Abdomen	gallbladder	nyongo
Abdomen	intestines, small	chango; utumbo mdogo
Abdomen	colon	utumbo mpana
Abdomen	rectum	mjiko
Abdomen	spleen	wengu; bandama
Abdomen	kidney (kidneys)	figo (mafigo)
Abdomen	urethra	mrija wa kutoa mkojo nje kutoka kibofu
Abdomen	ureter	mrija kutoka figo na kibofu cha mkojo
Abdomen	pancreas	kongosho
Abdomen	urinary bladder	kibofu cha mkojo
Abdomen	umbilicus	kitovu
Abdomen	umbilical cord	ukamba; kitovu
Pelvis	buttock (buttocks)	tako (matako)
Pelvis	vagina	uke
Pelvis	clitoris	kinembe
Pelvis	uterus (womb)	mfuko la uzazi
Pelvis	anus	mkundu
Pelvis	penis	uume; mboo
Pelvis	scrotum/testicle	pumbu; kende
Pelvis	pelvis (groin)	fupayonga (kinena)
Pelvis	hip	nyonga
Lower limbs	femur/thigh	paja
Lower limbs	leg (legs)	mguu (miguu)

51

Body parts	English	Swahili
Lower limbs	knee	goti
Lower limbs	patella	pia ya mguu; kilegesambwa
Lower limbs	lower leg	chini ya mguu
Lower limbs	shin	muundi
Lower limbs	calf	shavu la mguu
Lower limbs	ankle	kifundo cha mguu
Lower limbs	achilles' tendon	Ukano wa kisigino
Lower limbs	heel	kisigino
Lower limbs	foot (feet)	wayo
Lower limbs	big toe	gumba
Lower limbs	toe (toes)	kidole cha mguu (vidole cha mguu)
Lower limbs	toenail	ukucha wa kidole cha mguu

English-Swahili: abdomen-coronary

English	Swahili
abdomen *The portion of the body bordered by the diaphragm and the pelvis.*	tumbo
abdomen, lower	chini ya tumbo
abdominal girth *Waist circumference.*	tumbo kiwiliwili
abdominocentesis *Puncturing of the abdominal wall for drainage purposes.*	kuondolewa kwa maji kutoka tumbo kutumia sindano
abdominoperineal *Referring to the abdominal and perineal region.*	-a tumbo na msamba
abduct *To move a body part away from the body.*	sogeza kwa upande
aberrant *Different than normal.*	mapotofu
abnormal	kigego
ABO system *The system using human blood antigens to determine blood type.*	aina ya damu
abortion (miscarriage) *Premature expulsion of the fetus from the uterus.*	kutoa mimba
abortion, inevitable *Presence of cervical dilation or ruptured membranes in a pregnancy where the baby is not viable.*	kuepukika kuharibika kwa mimba
above	juu, juu ya
abrasion *Superficial skin injury.*	mkwaruzo
abrupt *Suddenly or hastily.*	ghafla
abscess *A localized collection of pus.*	jipu (majipu)
absence of	kukosekana kwa
absolute	kabisa
abstain, to *To give up or to stop.*	kuzira au epuka
abuse (sexual abuse)	unyanyasaji
accelerate *(To accelerate the healing process).*	kuongeza kasi ya
access *Means of entry.*	njia ya kuingia
accessory *Complimentary or concomitant.*	nyongeza
accident	tukio (matukio); ajali
accommodation *A term used to describe the ability of the eye to adjust to various distances.*	uwezo wa jicho kuzoea kuona tofauti katika umbali
accomplish, to *Achieve.*	kutimiza
according to	kulingana na
acephalous *A absence of a head.*	pasipo kichwa
acetabulum *The cup-shaped cavity with which the head of the femur articulates.*	kikombe cha nyonga
ache *A mild pain*	umivu
achieve, to *To complete something one was striving for.*	kufikia
Achilles tendon *Also called calcaneal tendon; tendon with insertion at the gasrocnemius & soleus into the tuberosity of the calcaneus*	mshipa wa kisigino
acid *Substance with a pH less than 7.*	asidi
acne *Inflamed or infected sebaceous glands.*	chunusi
acoustic *Referring to the auditory system.*	akimaanisha mfumo wa kusikia

53

English	Swahili
acquaint, to *To make someone familiar with something.*	kuwafahamisha
Acquired Immunodeficiency Syndrome (AIDS) *Presence of an AIDS defining illness or having a CD4 of less than 200/mm3.*	ukimwi
acromegaly *Hyperplasia of the nose, jaw, fingers and toes.*	upanuzi wa mifupa ya miguu na mikono na uso
acromioclavicular joint *Referring to the junction of the acromion and clavicle. (shoulder)*	fuzi
acute *Abrupt onset.*	papo hapo
Adam's apple *A prominence on the anterior neck caused by the thyroid cartilage of the larynx.*	kikoromeo
add, to *To count.*	kuongeza
addiction *An abnormal dependency.*	uzoevu; mraibu
adduction *To bring toward the midline.*	kuleta kuelekea katikati
adenitis *The inflammation of a gland.*	kuvimba tezi
adenopathy *Generally referring to a condition of the lymphatic glands.*	ugonjwa wa matezi
adequate *Sufficient.*	kutosha
adherence *To stick to something figuratively or literally.*	uzingatiaji
adjust, to *To modify a plan.*	kurekebisha
adjustment *A modification of a plan.*	marekebisho
adjuvant *Term used to describe the medical treatment after initial therapy, as in adjuvant radiation therapy after initial chemotherapy.*	itakayosaidia
admission (to hospital) *To be admitted.*	pata kitanda
adolescence	ujana
adult *Generally considered a person over 18 years old.*	watu wazima
adverse effect *In reference to medication use, it is an undesirable consequence of the drug.*	mbaya ya athari
advise, to *To give counsel.*	kushauri
afebrile *Absence of fever.*	kukosa homa
affect *The expression of emotions or feelings.*	kuathiri
affinity *To have a natural liking for.*	mshikamano
after-pains *The pain experienced after childbirth caused by uterine contractions.*	zingizi
after-taste *The sensation of a prolonged savor following eating/ drinking.*	baada ya ladha
afterbirth *The tissue expelled after the birth of a child that includes the placenta and allied membranes.*	kondo ya nyuma
age *Length of life.(old age)*	umri (umri mkubwa)
aggression *Violent or hostile behavior.*	uchokozi
agitation *A state of extreme emotional disturbance.*	fadhaa
agony *Anguish or torment.*	maumivu makai; uchungu
agoraphobia *The fear of being in a large open space.*	uoga wa kutangamana na watu
agreement *Accordance in opinion or feeling.*	makubaliano
ague *A term used to describe recurrent fever and shivering typically associated with malaria.*	homa na kutetemeka; kitapo
AIDS *Acquired Immunodeficiency Syndrome*	UKIMWI

English	Swahili
air	hewa
air hunger *The sensation of shortness of breath.*	hamu kubwa ya kupumua lakini kutokuwa na uwezo
akathisia *A condition exhibited by motor restlessness and inability to sit quietly.*	kutotulia
albino *A person who lacks pigment in the eyes, skin and hair.*	zeruzeru
alcohol *Ethanol or ethyl alcohol.*	pombe
alcoholism *An addiction to alcohol.*	pombe madawa ya kulevya
alert *Being in a watchful, ready state.*	tahadhari
alexia *Inability to read due to a central brain lesion.*	ukosefu wa uwezo wa kusoma kutokana na ugonjwa wa ubongo
algid *cold*	baridi
alkalosis *A condition in which the pH is increased.*	hali inayoletwa na kupungua kwa asidi mwilini
allergen *Compound that causes an allergic reaction.*	Dutu hii ambayo inaweza kusababisha mmenyuko mzio
allergy *An immune response by the body to a compound it is hypersensitive to.*	mzio
alleviate, to	kupunguza
alopecia *The absence of hair in areas where it normally exists.*	nywele kupotea
alteration *The process of change or modification.*	mabadiliko
Alzheimer's disease *A dementia of unknown cause or pathogenesis.*	ugonjwa wa Alzheimer
ambidextrous *Ability to use both hands equal ability.*	uwezo wa kutumia mikono yote miwili kwa wepesi
ambulance *A vehicle that carries the sick or injured.*	gari kwamba hubeba wagonjwa au kujeruhiwa
ambulation *Relating to walking.*	kutembea
amenorrhea *The absence of menses.*	ukosefu wa mzunguko wa hedhi
amentia *The absence of mental ability.*	ukosefu wa uwezo wa kiakili
amnesia *The inability to remember past events.*	kupoteza kumbukumbu
amniocentesis *Transabdominal aspiration of amniotic fluid.*	matumizi ya sindano ya kuondoa maji kutoka tumboni
amnion *The membrane lining the placenta which produces the amniotic fluid.*	mfuko wa ya mimba
amniotic fluid *The fluid surrounding the fetus.*	maji yanayozunguka kijusi; ugiligili ya amnioni (kuzunguka kijusi wakati wa mimba)
amount *The total or the aggregate.*	kiasi
amputation *Typically referring to the surgical removal of a limb.*	upasuaji kuondolewa kwa mkono au mguu
anal fistula *An opening in the skin that tracts to the anal canal thus causing some fecal material to leak from the opening in the skin.*	nasuri ya haja kubwa
anal *Near or referring to the anus.*	mkundu
analgesia *The absence of pain.*	kutokuwepo kwa maumivu
analgesic *A medication used to remove pain.*	dawa kutumika kuondoa maumivu

55

English	Swahili
analogous *To resemble or be similar to.*	sawa
anaphylaxis *An exaggerated response to a foreign substance.*	majibu ya chumvi na dutu
anastomosis *Surgical formation of a connection between two previously separate parts.*	Upasuaji uhusiano kati ya vipande viwili tofauti za mwili
anatomy *The study of body structure.*	utafiti wa muundo wa mwili
anemia *Lower than normal red blood cell count.*	upungufu wa damu
anencephaly *The congenital absence of the cranial vault and cerebral hemispheres.*	ukosefu wa ubongo
anesthesia *Loss of sensation.*	ganzi; nusukaputi
anesthetic *A chemical that produces anesthesia.*	matumizi ya dawa ya kufanya mtu usingizi wakati wa upasuaji
aneurysm *A condition exhibited by the dilatation of the walls of an artery or vein to form a blood-filled sac.*	kivimbe cha mshipa wa damu
angina pectoris *Exercise induced myocardial ischemia.*	kifua maumivu yanayosababishwa na mtiririko maskini damu
angioedema *Also called angioneurotic edema, it is caused by a histamine reaction. It can produce welts in mild cases but in severe cases can cause swelling of the lips and tongue.*	kufura kwa upande wa ndani wa midomo, kinywa na sehemu zinginezo za njia ya pumzi
anguish *Significant mental or physical pain.*	dhiki
anisomelia *Unequal size of arms or legs.*	kifua maumivu yanayosababishwa na mtiririko maskini damu
ankle *The area of the ankle joint.*	kifundo cha mguu
ankle edema or dependent edema *Extracellular fluid volume noted by swelling or pitting.*	kifundo cha mguu wa mapafu
ankle joint *The articulation of the tibia/fibula and talus.*	kifundo cha mguu wa pamoja
ankle swelling *Enlargement of the ankle region with or without pitting.*	kifundo cha mguu uvimbe
anomia *Inability to name or recognize familiar objects.*	ukosefu wa uwezo wa kutambua vitu ukoo
anorchous *The absence of testicles.*	ukosefu wa korodani
anorexia *The loss of appetite.*	kupoteza hamu ya kula
anosmia *Lack of the sense of smell.*	ukosefu wa uwezo wa harufu
anovulatory cycle *A menstrual cycle in which no ovum is released.*	bila kuachilia yai
anoxia *Reduced oxygen levels in body tissues.*	kupunguza oksijeni ngazi katika damu
antenatal *Refers to events before birth.*	muda kabla ya kujifungua
anterior *Toward the front.*	mbele
anthelmintic *An agent used to destroy worms.*	dawa kuharibu minyoo ya tumbo
anthrax *An infectious disease caused by Bacillus anthracis; there are cutaneous, inhalation and gastrointestinal syndromes.*	kimeta
anti-diarrheal *Medication used to treat diarrhea.*	pingamizi la kuhara
anti-inflammatory *Medication used to reduce inflammation.*	dawa kutumika kupunguza uvimbe
antibiotic *A medication that inhibits or kills microorganisms.*	dawa kutumika kutibu vya magonjwa

56

English	Swahili
antibody *A protein that combines with and counteracts foreign substances.*	zindiko
anticoagulant *Medication used to inhibit coagulation.*	dawa kutumika nyembamba ya damu
anticonvulsant *Medication used to treat seizures.*	dawa kutumika kutibu kifafa
antidepressant *Medication used to treat depression.*	dawa kutumika kutibu huzuni
antidote *A medication that neutralizes a toxin.*	dawa kutumika kukabiliana na sumu; kiuasumu
antiemetic *A medication used to control nausea.*	pingamizi la kutapika
antimalarial *Medication used to treat malaria.*	dawa kutumika kutibu malaria
antimigraine *Medication used to treat headaches.*	dawa kutumika kutibu maumivu ya kichwa
antipruritic *Medication used to treat pruritus.*	dawa kutumika kutibu kuwasha
antipyretic *Medication used to treat fever.*	dawa zinazotumika kutibu homa
antitussive *Medication used to diminish a cough.*	dawa kutumika kupunguza kikohozi
antivenin *An antitoxin formulated for various types of snake bites.*	dawa ya kuharibu nguvu ya sumu ya nyoka
anuria *The lack of urine excretion.*	ukosefu wa mkojo
anus *The body opening distal to the rectum.*	mkundu
anxiety *Nervousness or unease.*	wasiwasi
anxious *Experiencing nervousness or unease.*	kuwa wa wasiwasi
aorta *The large artery originating at the left ventricle and going to the pelvis where it bifurcates.*	mshipa mkubwa wa damu wa upande wa kushoto wa moyo
aortic valve *The valve situated between the left ventricle and the aorta.*	kilango cha arteri kubwa
apart *Separated by a distance.*	mbali
apathy *Lack of interest in one's environment or indifference.*	ubaridi
apex *The highest point of something.*	kilele
aphagia *The lack of eating.*	ukosefu wa kula
aphasia *Diminished ability to communicate via speech or writing.*	ukosefu wa uwezo wa kusema
aphonia *The loss of voice.*	kupoteza sauti
apnea *Absence of respiration.*	ukosefu wa kupumua
apoplexy *Extravasation of blood within an organ. For example, neonatal apoplexy is consistent with intracranial hemorrhage.*	kiharusi
appearance *The way someone looks or presents.*	kuonekana
appendectomy *Surgical excision of the appendix.*	upasuaji kuondoa kibole
appendicitis *Inflammation of the appendix.*	kidoletumbo
appendix *An appendage of the cecum.*	kibole
appetite *A desire to eat.*	hamu ya chakula
application *The forms one fills out to obtain a grant.*	maombi
applicator *A device used to apply a topical medication.*	kifaa kutumika kuomba dawa
appointment *A previously scheduled time to see a person.*	utezi
apprehensive *A fear that something unpleasant will happen.*	wasiwasi
approval *Accepting something as satisfactory.*	idhini
approximate, to *To bring together, as in wound margins.*	kuleta kishindo jeraha pamoja

English	Swahili
approximately *Nearly but not completely.*	takriban
aptitude *A natural talent for something.*	vipaji asili
aptyalism *Diminished or absence of saliva.*	ukosefuu wa mate
aqueous humor *The fluid between the cornea and lens, anterior to the globe.*	maji katika sehemu ya mbele ya jicho
arachnodactyly *A condition exhibited by abnormally long and slender fingers.*	kidole kwa muda mrefu mwembamba
arachnoid *Refers to that which resembles a spider web.*	kipande cha katikati kwenye zile ngozi tatu zifunikazo ubongo
argue, to *To debate or reason. (quarrel)*	kujadili
arm *One of two upper extremities.*	mkono
armpit *A common term for axilla.*	kwapa
around *On every side of.*	karibu
arrhythmia *An abnormal heart rhythm.*	yasiyo ya kawaida
arteriosclerosis *Hardening and thickening of arterial walls.*	hali ya arteri kupata ugumu, kusongana na kupoteza uwezo wa kunyumbuka au kurefuka
arteritis *Inflammation of an artery.*	kiwasho cha mshipa mkubwa
artery *Vessel that carries oxygenated blood from the heart to the periphery.*	mshipa mkubwa
arthritis *Joint inflammation.*	ugua mifupa
artificial *Not natural produced.*	bandia
ascaricide *Agent that destroys ascaris.*	dawa ambayo kuharibu minyoo ya tumbo
ascaris *A nematode from genus intestinal lumbricoid parasite, also called round worm.*	aina ya minyoo ya tumbo
ascertain, to *Synonym of "to determine".*	kuamua
ascites *Serous fluid in the abdominal cavity.*	istiska
asepsis *Lack of infection.*	ukosefu wa maambukizi ya
asleep *To be in a dormant or inactive state.*	amelala
aspermia *Absence of sperm.*	ukosefu wa shahawa
asphyxia *A condition exhibited by a lack of oxygen and subsequent loss of consciousness or death.*	kukosekana hewa
aspiration biopsy *Removal of fluid from a cavity for pathologic analysis.*	kuondolewa kwa maji ya mwili kwa kutumia sindano ya kutathmini kwa ajili ya ugonjwa
assessment *An medical evaluation.*	matibabu tathmini
assistance *The act of helping.*	huduma
asterixis *Commonly known as a flapping tremor, it is characterized by involuntary jerking movements of the hands and is seen commonly in hepatic encephalopathy.*	shituko harakati ya mikono
asthenia *Diminished strength and energy.*	udhaifu wa mwili
asthma *An inflammatory disease of the lungs noteworthy because of reversible airway obstruction.*	pumu
astringent *An agent causing contraction of the skin.*	kutuliza nafsi
asymmetry *Lack of symmetry.*	ukosefu wa ulinganifu
asymptomatic *The absence of symptoms.*	ukosefu wa dalili
at random *Occurring by chance alone.*	shaghala

58

English	Swahili
ataxia *Lack of muscular coordination.*	Ukosefu wa uratibu wa misuli
athetosis *An involuntary symptom exhibited by continuous slow, writhing movements, mostly in the hands.*	songo harakati cha mikono
athlete's foot *Common term for tinea pedis.*	nyungunyungu
atrium *Referring to a chamber used as an entrance, as in the entrance to the heart.*	sehemu ya uu ya kila nusu ya moyo
atrophy *A diminution in the size of a part.*	uliopooza misuli
atypical *Not usual.*	usio wa kawaida
auditory agnosia *Caused by a temporal lobe lesion, it is characterized by inability to recognize sounds as words.*	kutokuwa na uwezo wa kutambua sauti kama maneno
auricle *The external portion of the ear.*	sehemu ya nje ya sikio
auscultation *The act of listening to sounds emanating from the body.*	kusikiliza kwa msaada wa kifaa cha matibabu
autopsy *Examination of a body post-mortem in an attempt to determine cause of death.*	uchunguzi baada ya kifo
availability *A person or thing that is available.*	upatikanaji
available *Attainable, obtainable.*	inapatikana
avoidable *That which can be stopped or inhibited.*	zaweza kuepukwa
awakening *The state of being conscious.*	kuamka
away from *Separated from.*	mbali na
axilla *The hollow beneath the arm.*	kwapa
baby *A newborn.*	mchanga
baby-scale *A device used to weigh an infant.*	mtoto-wadogo
back pain *Discomfort on the dorsal surface of the torso.*	maumivu ya mgongo
bacteria *Plural for any organism of the order Eubacteriales.*	kijimea
balanitis *Inflammation of the glans of the penis.*	kuvimba katika mwisho wa uume
balm *A topical medical preparation.*	zeri
bandage *A strip of gauze used to immobilize or support.*	bendeji
bandage tied to a circumcised penis	alfafa
basin *A small bowl used for washing.*	bakuli
basophil *A polymorphonuclear granulocyte.*	besofili
bear, to *To endure or resist.*	kupinga
bear, to *To give birth to a child.*	kuzaa
bearing down *As in during labor.*	kuzaa chini
beat *As in heart beat.*	kupiga cha moyo
bed rest *A medical order requiring one to stay in bed.*	kitanda mapumziko
bedbug Cimex lectularius. *A small insect that is parasitic and hides in clothing or bedding.*	kunguni
bedpan *A metal or plastic vestibule one sits on while in bed to defecate.*	sufuria kitanda
bedridden *Term used to indicate one is so ill they cannot get out of bed.*	kitandani
beds *A mattress resting on a frame. (plural)*	vitanda
bee sting *A piercing from a bee.*	nyuki
beforehand *In advance or previously.*	kabla ya
behavior disorder *An abnormal mental state.*	tabia machafuko

59

English	Swahili
belch *Eructation.*	mbweu
Bell's palsy *Unilateral facial paralysis related to dysfunction of the seventh cranial nerve.*	moja moja usoni kupooza (neva ya fuvu tatizo)
below *Under.*	chini ya
benign *Not harmful.*	hafifu
bereavement *The sorrow one feels with the loss of a loved one.*	msiba
best *Optimal or ideal.*	bora
beyond *On the farther side.*	zaidi ya
biased *Prejudiced.*	upendeleo
bilateral *Referring to both sides.*	za mwili
bile *An alkaline fluid secreted by the liver to aid digestion.*	nyongo
bile ducts *The structures that are conduits for passage of bile from the liver and gallbladder to the duodenum.*	mrija wa nyongo
Bilharzia *Historical name of a genus of flukes or nematodes now known as Schistosoma.*	kichocho
bill *A financial statement that indicates how much one owes.*	bili
biology *The study of living organisms.*	biolojia
birth *The process of bearing offspring from the uterus.*	uzazi
birth control *Any method of limiting contraception.*	uzazi wa majira
birth defect *A congenital anomaly.*	kuzaliwa makosa
bistoury; scalpel *A surgical knife.*	koleo
bitter (taste) *Having a harsh, unpleasant taste.*	chungu
black *Referring to the color, as in the color of coal.*	rangi nyeusi
black stools *Common term for melena.*	nyeusi kinyesi
blackout *Common term for loss of consciousness.*	kuzirai
blackwater fever *A term used to describe the fever associated with malaria when the urine is reddish-black.*	malaria (mkojo ni rangi nyekundu-nyeusi)
bladder, urinary *Vestibule for urine prior to being expelled via the urethra.*	kibofu cha mkojo
bleed *Loss of blood.*	tokwa na damu
blemish *A small mark on one's skin.*	doa
blepharitis *Inflammation of the eyelids.*	mchochota wa kope; kikope
blepharospasm *A spasm of the orbicularis oculi muscle that causes closure of the eyelid.*	kipindupindu ya misuli kwamba ni kutumika kwa karibu jicho
blind person *Person with absence of sight.*	kipofu
blindness *Absence of visual perception.*	upofu
blink, to *To open and close the eyelid rapidly.*	kupepesa (macho)
blister *Common term for bulla.*	lengelenge
bloated *Sensation of having an abnormally large amount of air in the viscera.*	riahi
blood *Plasma containing erythrocytes, leukocytes and platelets.*	damu
blood alcohol level *A quantitative measurement of the amount of alcohol in the blood.*	damu pombe ngazi
blood cells *A common term that does not differentiate between erythrocyte or leukocyte.*	selidamu
blood clot *A mass of coagulated blood.*	donge la damu
blood grouping *Testing blood to determine which type should be used for transfusion.*	aina ya damu

60

English	Swahili
blood pressure *Written as the measurement in mmHg at the time of systole of the left ventricle over the time of diastole.*	msukumo wa damu; shinikizo la damu
blood stream *Common term or the arterial or venous systems.*	mshipa wa damu
blood type *Determined and listed in the ABO system.*	aina damu
blood-letting *The removal of blood from a patient with the thought it would cure or prevent disease.*	kuumika
blue *A color between green and violet.*	rangi ya buluu
blunt *Having a flat or rounded end.*	butu
blurred vision *Low visual acuity. (fuzzy vision)*	kiwaa (kinyenyezi)
blurt out, to *To speak without considering the repercussions.*	boboka
blush, to *To have an increased volume of blood flow to one's face causing a red tint to the skin.*	haya usoni
body surface area *Dubois formula is: (weight in kilograms)to the 0.425th power x (height in centimeters) to the 0.725th power x 0.007184.*	mwili uso eneo
body *The physical structure of a person.*	mwili
body weight *Relative mass as measured in kilograms or pounds.*	uzito wa mwili
boil *Small abscess or furuncle.*	jipu
bone *Skeletal tissue formed by osteoblasts.*	mfupa
bone marrow *The soft material filling the cavity of bones.*	uboho
born, to be *Being present as a result of birth.*	zaliwa
bottle *A container used for the storage of liquids.*	chupa
bow-legged person	matege
brace *A splint.*	banzi
brace, to *Application of a splint.*	maombi ya banzi
brachial plexus *A cluster of nerves coming off the last four cervical and first thoracic spinal nerves form the nerve supply the the chest and arms.*	brachial mishipa ya fahamu
bradycardia *Lower than normal cardiac rate measured in beats per minute.*	mfupi upana fuvu
brain *A common term for cerebrum.*	ubongo
brain death *Cessation of cerebral functioning.*	ubongo kifu
brain stem *An organ that consists of the medulla oblongata, pons and midbrain.*	sehemu ya ubongo inayounganisha ubongo na uti wa mgongo
break *A common term for a fracture in a bone.*	kuvunjika
breast *Mammary tissue including the areola.*	ziwa
breast feeding *The process of giving milk to a baby via the nipple.*	kunyonyesha
breath *One respiration.*	pumzi
breath sounds *The noise heard upon auscultation with a stethoscope.*	pumzi sauti
breath test (for alcohol) *A check of alcohol level by testing exhaled air.*	jaribio la pumzi kwa ajili ya pombe
breech birth *Delivery with the feet or buttocks coming first.*	tako kuzaliwa
breech presentation *Position of the feet or buttocks near the cervix.*	hali ya mtoto kutangulia na matako anapozaliwa
bright *Giving out a lot of light.*	mkali

English	Swahili
bring, to *To carry or transport something.*	kuleta
brisk *Rapid or fast.*	hima
broken (arm) *Fracture of the arm.*	kuvunjwa mkono
bromidrosis *Foul smelling perspiration.*	mchafu kunusa jasho
bronchiole *A small branch that a bronchus divides into.*	vinjia vidogo vya hewa kwenya mapufu
bronchitis *Inflammation of the mucous membranes of the bronchioles that causes bronchospasm and cough.*	mkamba
bronchus *The major air channels that bifurcate from the distal trachea.*	mojawapo ya zile njia mbili kubwa za hewa kutoka kwenye pipa la hewa
brow presentation *The term used to describe which part of the body (forehead) is being delivered first in childbirth.*	paji la uso ni sehemu kuwasilisha wakati anapozaliwa
brown *Coffee-colored.*	rangi ya kahawia
bruise *Common term for ecchymosis.*	chubuko
bubo *An inflamed, swollen lymph node in the axilla or inguinal region.*	jipu la mtoki
bubonic plague *A form of plague exhibited by the formation of buboes.*	tauni ya majipu
buccal *Referring to the cheek.*	shavu
bug *Insect.*	mdudu
bulge *A protuberance on a flat surface.*	mbenuko
burn *An injury caused by exposure to heat.*	choma
burst, to *To rupture.*	tumbuka
buttocks (buttock) *The bilateral region covering the gluteal muscles.*	matako (tako); makalio
cachexia *Generalized weakness and severe wasting.*	kali kukonda
cadaver *A dead body.*	maiti
calcaneus *Commonly called the heel bone.*	mfupa wa kisigino
calcium *A chemical element that is an essential component in teeth and bone.*	kalsiamu
calculus *A stone of minerals that can lead to the blockage of the bile duct or ureters.*	kijiwe na mkusanyiko wa chokaa mwilini
calf *Muscles of the posterior portion of the lower leg.*	shavu la mguu
callosity *Callus; thickened hardened skin.*	sugu
cancel, to *To stop or revoke.*	kutangua
cancer; carcinoma *A disease of uncontrolled abnormal cell growth.*	kansa; saratani
candle *A cylindrical piece of wax with a central wick.*	mshumaa
canine teeth *Located between the incisors and premolars.*	jino chongo
canker sore *An ulceration, usually of the mouth or lips.*	donda kidonda
capillary *A vessel that connects arterioles to venules.*	mishipa midogu ya damu ambapo mabadilishano ya hewa kati ya damu na viungo vya mwili hutokeo
capsule *Medication in the form of a capsule.*	tembe
caput *The head.*	kichwa
carbon monoxide poisoning *This tasteless, odorless gas causes constitutional symptoms but can lead to death upon inhalation.*	sumu monoksidi kaboni

English	Swahili
cardiac *Referring to the heart.*	moyo
cardiac arrest *Cessation of function of the heart.*	kukoma kwa uwezo wa moyo kupiga
cardiopulmonary resuscitation *Use of artificial means to support respiration and circulation.*	moyo-mapafu kufufuliwa
cardiovascular *Referring to the heart or circulatory system.*	inayohusiana na moyo, mishipa ya damu na damu
caregiver *A person who provides care to another.*	mlezi
caries *Referring to decay or death of a tooth.*	kuoza kwa jino
carotid *Referring to the large artery on each side of the neck.*	kubwa ateri katika shingo
carpopedal spasm *A spasm of the carpus and the foot.*	kukazana kwa misuli kwenye miguu na mikono
cartilage *Firm, relatively non-vascular connective tissue.*	gegedu
cast; plaster cast *Use of plaster of paris to immobilize an extremity.*	plasta
castration *Excision of the gonads.*	uhasi
casualty *A person who is killed or seriously injured.*	majeruhi
cataract *An opacity of an eye lens or the capsule.*	mtoto wa jicho
catarrh *Inflammation of a mucous membrane.*	kuvimba utando wa kamasi; mafua
catch a cold *To come down with a viral upper respiratory tract infection.*	kuendeleza mafua
catheter *A flexible tube inserted into the body.*	kifaa kama mrija kinachotiwa mwilini ili kutoa au kutia vitu vya aina ya majimaji
caudal *Referring to a cauda.*	mkia
cavity *Pouch or chamber.*	mvungu
center *A point equidistant from all sides.*	kati
central nervous system (CNS) *The brain and spinal cord.*	ubongo na uti wa mgongo
cephalic *Towards the head.*	kuelekea kichwa
cerebellum *The part of the brain in the posterior portion of the skull that controls muscle coordination and movement.*	nyuma sehemu ya ubongo
cerebrospinal fluid (CSF) *The fluid between the pia mater and arachnoid membrane.*	ugiligili ya ubongo na uti wa mgongo (kuzunguka ubongo na uti wa mgongo)
cerebrovascular accident (stroke) *A decrease in level of consciousness and paralysis caused by a cerebrovascular thrombosis, hemorrhage or vasospasm.*	kuzuiwa kwa damu kufikia sehemu fulani za ubongo
cerumen impaction *External ear canal full of wax resulting in hearing loss until the impaction is removed.*	sikio mfereji imefungwa na nta
cerumen *Waxy substance found normally in the external ear canals.*	nta ya sikio
cervix uteri *The narrow end of the uterus.*	sehemu ya chini iliyo nyembamba katika chungu cha mtoto
cesarean section *Incision of the abdominal and uterine walls in order to deliver a fetus when natural delivery is not possible.*	upasuaji wa kutoa mtoto
chancre *The initial ulcer that is seen with primary syphilis.*	kwanza kidonda ya kaswende
check for, to	na kuangalia kwa

63

English	Swahili
cheek *Lateral facial tissue.*	shavu
cheekbone	kitefute
chemotaxis *The response of an organism to chemical agents.*	kemotaksi
chemotherapy *Use of medication (chemical agents) in the treatment of disease. This term is commonly used to refer to the treatment of cancer patients with medication.*	tibakemikali
chest *Thorax.*	kifua
chest wall *Thoracic wall.*	kifua ukuta
chew, to *Masticate.*	kutafuna
chicken pox, varicella *A viral disease characterized by extremely pruritus blisters over the entire body.*	tekekuwanga
chigger *A parasitic mite of the genus Trombicula.*	tekenywa
child *A person aged 1 to 8 years old. (male, female)*	mtoto (kiume, kike)
childbirth *Parturition; the process of labor and delivery of an infant.*	uzazi wa mtoto
childhood *The time between infancy and puberty.*	utoto
chill *Sensation of coldness.*	mzizimo, baridi; kitapo
chin *Mentum; the anterior projection of the lower jaw.*	kidevu
choice *Selection or decision.*	uchaguzi
choke *To retch, cough or fight for breath.*	hulisonga
cholecystectomy *Surgical excision of the gallbladder.*	upasuaji kuondoa nyongo
cholecystitis *Inflammation of the gallbladder.*	kuvimba nyongo
cholera *An infectious disease exhibited by vomiting and diarrhea and caused by Vibrio cholerae.*	kipindupindu
cholesterol *A compound or its derivatives are found in cell membranes and precursors to hormones but high levels can cause atherosclerosis.*	kolesteroli
chronic *When referring to an illness, it means recurring or persistent.*	inayotokea pole pole, huchukua muda mrefu, isiyo ya ghafla
cicatrix (scar) *New tissue in a healed wound.*	kovu
cilia *The hairs growing on the eyelid or a motile extension of a cell surface.*	kama nywele
circadian *Referring to a 24 hour period.*	sikadiani
circumcision *Surgical excision of the foreskin.*	tohara; tahiri
circumference *The distance around an object or part.*	mduara
cirrhosis *A liver disease characterized by destruction of liver cells and increased connective tissue.*	ugonjwa wa ini
clavicle *A bone that articulates with the sternum and scapula.*	mtulinga
clear one's throat, to *To cough lightly in attempt to speak more clearly.*	wazi moja wa koo
clear *Transparent.*	wazi
clearance *The process of removing something.*	kibali
cleavage *A sharp division or demarcation.*	mwanya
cleft lip *A congenital abnormal opening of the lip.*	kitakapo mdomo
cleft palate *A congenital abnormal opening in the palate.*	kitakapo kaakaa
clinic *A building where patients are evaluated.*	zahanati
clitoris *A small erectile body in the anterosuperior aspect of the vulva.*	kisimi

English	Swahili
closed	kufungwa
clot *A thrombus or embolus.*	vilio
cluster headache *A unilateral, severe, recurrent headache.*	moja moja maumivu makali ya kichwa
coagulation *The formation of a clot.*	vilio
coccyx *The small bone formed by the natural fusion of rudimentary vertebrae.*	kifandugu
cochlea *The essential organ of hearing which is in a spiral form.*	mfereji wenye umbo la
cockroach *A beetle-like insect with long legs and antennae.*	kombamwiko
cognition *The process of acquiring thought or understanding.*	utambuzi
coitus *Sexual intercourse between members of the opposite sex.*	ngono
cold *Having a sense of being cold.*	baridi
cold sore *A perioral blister caused by herpes simplex.*	baridi sana
cold *Viral upper respiratory tract infection.*	mufua
colectomy *Surgical removal of part of the colon.*	upasuaji kuondolewa matumbo kubwa
colic *Acute abdominal pain.*	msokoto wa tumbo
colitis *Inflammation of the colon.*	kuvimba matumbo kubwa
collapse *A physical or mental breakdown.*	kuanguka
collarbone *Common term for the clavicle.*	mtulinga
colon *The portion of the large intestine that goes from the cecum to the rectum.*	kubwa ya matumbo
color blindness *The inability to distinguish colors.*	kutoweza kupambanua rangi tofauti
colostrum *The fluid secreted by the mammary glands a few days around parturition.*	kiamo
coma *A state of unconsciousness.*	hali ya kuzimia roho
comedone *The medical term (singular) for blackheads.*	kidutu
comment *A remark providing an opinion.*	maoni
common *That which is usual.*	kawaida
compatible *To coexist without problems.*	sambamba
compendium *A concise summary about a subject.*	maandishi
complaint *Grievance.*	malalaliko
compliance *The act of going along with a plan.*	kufuata
comply, to *Adhere to.*	kuzingatia
compound *A substance formed by covalent union of two or more atoms.*	unga dawa
comprehension *Understanding.*	ufahamu
concentric *Referring to circles or arcs that share the same center.*	senta
conception *The act of an egg being fertilized by sperm.*	kutunga mimba
concussion *Head trauma resulting in temporary loss of consciousness.*	mtikiso
condom *A covering for the penis or the vagina (female condom) used during sexual intercourse that is meant to reduce the chance of pregnancy or infection.*	kondomu
confabulation *The fabrication of experiences to compensate for memory loss.*	kupayuka maneno ovyo

65

English	Swahili
confidence *Self-assurance.*	kujiamini
confinement *As in confined to bed.*	kifungo
conflict *Dispute or disagreement.*	migogoro
confusion *Disorientation.*	machafuko
congenital *A disease or anomaly present from birth.*	tangu kuzaliwa
congenital syphilis *Passed to the child in utero, the child may have failure to thrive, fever and a flattened bridge of the nose.*	tangu kuzaliwa kaswende
congestive heart failure *A diminished cardiac output leading to passive engorgement.*	kukoma kwa moyo kutokana na marilio ya damu hali ya kujazuna
conjunctiva *The membrane that lines the eyelid.*	ngozi nyembamba inayofunika sehemu ya ndani ya macho
conjunctivitis *Inflammation of the conjunctiva.*	kiwasho ya ngozi nyembamba inayofunika sehemu ya nje ya jicho ndani ya kope
conscious *Being award and being able to respond to one's surroundings.*	kutanabahi
conservative *Control rather than elimination of a disease.*	kihafidhina
consistent *Compatible with something or congruous with.*	thabiti
constipation *A condition exhibited by difficulty in having a bowel movement due to hard stools.*	funga choo
constriction *Circumferential tightening*	mfinyo
contact *The touching of two bodies or a person who has been exposed to a contagious disease.*	kuwasiliana na
contagious *Description of a disease that can be spread by direct or indirect contact.*	kuambukiza
contaminate, to *To make impure by exposing to an polluted agent.*	kuchafua
content *What something is made up of.*	maudhui
contraceptive *A device or medication used to prevent pregnancy.*	uzazi wa mpango
contradictory *Two elements that are inconsistent.*	kupingana
contraindication *A situation in which two elements are inconsistent.*	utata
contusion *An area of broken capillaries in the skin causing discoloration; commonly called a bruise.*	chubuko
convenient *Opportune or well-timed.*	rahisi
convulsions *An involuntary series of tonic and clonic movements.*	mishtuko
cool *Chilly or cold.*	poa
cope, to *To deal with a difficult situation.*	kukabiliana
cord compression *Pressure being applied to the spinal cord.*	usiokuwa wa kawaida shinikizo kutumiwa na uti wa mgongo
cornea *The transparent segment located at the anterior part of the eye.*	konea
corneal transplant *Surgical replacement of a cornea with a donor cornea.*	upasuaji badala ya konea
coronary vessel *Referring to a coronary artery.*	mshipa unaopeleka damu kwenye misuli ya moyo

66

English-Swahili: corpulence-Hansen's

English	Swahili
corpulence *Fatness.*	ujazi
coryza *An acute condition exhibited by copious nasal discharge.*	kutokwa na makamasi mengi
cost *The fee or penalty.*	gharama
cotton wool *Raw cotton.*	pamba
cough *Forceful expulsion of air from the lungs.*	kikohozi
coughing fit *An episode of prolonged, forceful coughing.*	kukohoa kipindupindu
count, to *To determine a number.*	kuhesabu
cow's milk	maziwa ya ng'ombe
coxalgia *Pain in the hip.*	kiuno maumivu
crab louse *Phthirus pubis is formal name for a louse that infests pubic hair and causes intense itching.*	kaa chawa
cramp *A painful contraction of muscles.*	mpindanowa misuli
craniotomy *Surgical creation of a hole in the skull.*	upasuaji wa kuwashirikisha fuvu
craving *An unusually strong urge for something.*	tamaa
craw-craw *A pruritic papular skin eruption sometimes caused by Onchocerca.*	firigisi-firigisi
crepitus *A noise heard when one auscultates the lungs that is similar to the sound of rubbing hair between one's fingers.(1) It is also considered the sound of two broken bones rubbing together. (2)*	makelele au sauti za mifupa iliyovunjika hasa wakati inapokwaruzana (2)
crevice *A narrow opening.*	mwanya
cripple *A person with a physical disability; not used in polite society.*	kiwete
crisis *A turning point in the treatment of a disease.*	mgogoro
Crohn's disease *An inflammatory bowel disease.*	ugonjwa wa Crohn
croup *An acute laryngeal condition that is accompanied by a hoarse, barking cough.*	hali ya kikohozi gumio
cruciform *Shaped like a cross.*	umbo kama msalaba
crust *Dried serous exudate covering a wound.*	kavu rishai
crutch *Long metal or wooden stick used for support while walking.*	mkongojo
CSF *Abbreviation for cerebrospinal fluid.*	maji uti wa mgongo
cumulative effect *A consequence of successive additions.*	nyongeza athari
cuneiform *The three bones between the navicular bone and the metatarsals.*	mifupa midogo ya mguu
curative *A remedy capable of healing completely.*	tiba
cure *A remedy for a medical illness.*	kutiba
curettage *Removal of tissues from a cavity.*	ukwanguaji
curette *The instrument used during a curettage.*	ala ya kukombea
current *Flow or stream.*	mkondo au mtiririko
currently *Presently.*	sasa
cushion *A pillow or stuffed pad used to sit on.*	mto
cut *An incision.*	mtai

English	Swahili
cuticle *The dead skin at the base of the toenail or fingernail, also called the eponychium.*	ukaya wa ukucha
cyanosis *Bluish discoloration of the skin and mucous membranes.*	sainosisi
cyclical vomiting *Periods of recurrent vomiting with no apparent pathologic cause and the person has a normal state of health between the episodes.*	matumizi ya kawaida ya kuapika
cystic fibrosis *A congenital disorder exhibited by abnormal thick mucous which leads to problems in the intestines, pancreas and lungs.*	uvimbe wa nyuzi
cystitis *Inflammation of the urinary bladder.*	mchochota wa kibofu cha mkojo
dacryocystitis *Inflammation of a lacrimal sac.*	kiwasho wa kifuko cha machozi
dandruff *Dead skin found in the hair.*	mba
date of admission *Beginning date of hospitalization.*	tarehe ya kuingia hospitalini
date of birth	tarehe ya kuzaliwa
daughter	binti
dead, to be *Deceased. (dead person)*	kumata(mfu)
deadline *Cutoff date.*	tarhe ya mwisho
deaf *Absence of the sense of hearing. (deaf person)*	ziwi (kiziwi)
deaf-mute *Inability to hear or speak.*	mtu aliye kiziwi na bubu
deafness *Having impaired hearing.*	uziwi
death *The action of dying.*	mauti
debility *Physical weakness.*	udhaifu
debridement *Trimming the dead tissue adjacent to a wound.*	kuondoa tishu zenye madhara
decade *Ten years.*	muongo
decapitate, to *The physical separation of the head from the body.*	kimwili mgawanyo wa kichwa na mwili
deciduous teeth *The first teeth.*	awali ya meno
decline *As in a decrease in status or health.*	punguza
decrease *Becoming smaller or fewer.*	upungufu
decubitus *Laying flat in bed or dorsal decubitus. (lateral decubitus is flat and on one's side)*	kuwekwa gorofa katika kitanda
decubitus ulcer *A wound caused by laying in one position for too long; also referred to as a pressure ulcer.*	kidonda kutoka kuwekewa gorofa katika kitanda
deep *Having significant depth.*	kina
deep vein thrombosis (DVT) *A blood clot that forms within a vein, typically in the lower extremities.*	kina cha mshipa donge
deer tick *Ixodes scapularis.*	kulungu kupe
defecation *The discharge of feces from the rectum.*	enda choo; enda mavi
defect *A shortcoming or imperfection.*	ila
deficiency *Insufficiency or deficit.*	upungufu
deformity *A malformation or imperfection.*	kilema
deglutition *The process of swallowing.*	kumeza
dehydration *The status of having a decrease in total body water.*	upungufu wa maji mwilini
delirium *An acute mental state exhibited by altered thought processes and restlessness.*	payo

68

English	Swahili
delirium tremens *A condition seen when alcohol is withdrawn which is exhibited by restlessness, hallucinations and tremors.*	payo mitikisiko
delivery *The process of giving birth. (forceps delivery)*	kuzaa (kujifungua kusaidiwa kwa koleo)
delusion *A belief that is contradictory to rational thought.*	udanganyifu
demarcation *Having a fixed boundary.*	kuwa mipaka ya kudumu
dementia *A chronic brain disorder exhibited by memory loss, personality changes and faulty reasoning.*	wazimu
dengue *A mosquito-borne viral disease exhibited by fever and joint pain.*	mbu yanayotokana na ugonjwa wa homa na maumivu
density *The denseness of an object.*	wiani
dental *Referring to teeth.*	meno
dental caries *Decay of teeth.*	kuoza kwa jino
dentist *A professional capable of treating diseases of the teeth and gums.*	daktari wa meno; tabibumeno; mhazigimeno
denture *A frame that holds artificial teeth.*	meno bandia
deny, to *To reject or repudiate.*	kukana
depressed *Melancholy.*	ghamu; soda
depression *A medical condition exhibited by profound despondency.*	mfadhaiko; usononi
deprivation *The lack of a necessity.*	kunyimwa
dermatitis *Non-specific inflammation of the skin.*	kuvimba wa ngozi
dermis *The "true skin" that lies beneath the epidermis.*	ngozi ya kwanza ya juu
descending *Moving toward the inferior portion.*	kushuka
desiccation *The act of drying up.*	ukaushaji
despite *Notwithstanding.*	licha ya
deterioration *Worsening in one's medical condition.*	kuzorota
detrimental *Harmful.*	mabaya
deviation *Away from the norm.*	kupotoka
diabetes insipidus *Caused by a deficiency in vasopressin, it is exhibited by great thirst and large volume urine output (and normal blood sugar).*	ugonjwa ulioonyeshwa na kiu kubwa sana na mkojo
diabetes mellitus *A disease exhibited by a deficiency of the pancreatic hormone insulin.*	ugonjwa ya sukari
diaphoretic *Exhibited by profuse perspiration.*	jasho mengi
diaphragm *The muscular separation between the thoracic and abdominal cavities.*	kiwambo cha moyo
diarrhea *Increase in frequency and a loose consistency of the stools.*	harisho
diarrhea, to have *(verb) The act of having diarrhea.*	kuhara, kuendesha
die, to *To stop living, to expire.*	kufa; kufariki
diet *The kinds of food a person eats.*	ulaji
differential diagnosis *A list of possible alternative diagnoses for a patient who is ill.*	orodha ya ugunduzi inawezekana
digestion *The process of enzymatic breakdown of food in the alimentary canal.*	kuvunjika kwa chakula katika matumbo
digit *Finger.*	kidole
dilatation *The process of becoming wider or larger.*	panua

69

dilator *An instrument that dilates.*	kipanulio
dilution *The process of making a weaker solution.*	uzimuaji
diphtheria *A contagious bacterial disease characterized by a grey membrane on the pharynx along with respiratory or cutaneous symptoms; caused by Corynebacterium diphtheriae.*	dondakoo
diplegia *The paralysis of both arms or both legs.*	kupooza kwa mbili yamefika
diplopia *Double vision.*	mara mbili ya maono
dipsomania *Compulsion to drink alcoholic beverages.*	tamaa kubwa ya ulevi
dirty *Unclean.*	chafu
disability *Decreased or impaired mental or physical ability.*	kutojiweza; ulemavu
disappearance *An instance of something/someone gone missing.*	upotevu
discharge date *The day a patient is released from the hospital.*	tarehe ya kuondoka hospitali
discharge, ear *Otic secretions.*	kinyaa cha masikio
discharge, nasal *Nasal secretions.*	kinyaa cha pua
discharge, postpartum vaginal *The secretions noted after delivery.*	uke kinyaa (baada ya kujifungua)
discharge, vaginal *Vaginal secretions.*	uke kinyaa
discomfort *A feeling of physical or mental unease.*	adha
discrete *Separate and distinct.*	tofauti na tofauti
disease *Malady or disorder.*	maradhi; ugonjwa
disease outcome *The response obtained from treatment.*	ugonjwa matokeo
disequilibrium *The absence of stability.*	ukosefu wa msawazo
disinfectant *A substance that kills bacteria.*	dawa ya kuondoa au kuua viini vya magonjwa
dislocation *The displacement of a bone when referring to an articulation. (sprain, dislocate, startle)*	mshtuko; kuathiriwa kwa uhusiano/ushirikiano wa kawaida wa kiungo
disorder *Impairment.*	ugonjwa wa
disorientation *Mental confusion.*	kuchanganyikiwa
displacement *Movement from normal position.*	makazi yao
disrobe, to *To remove clothing.*	kuondoa nguo
dissemination *To be spread or dispersed widely.*	usambazaji
distal *Situated away from the center of the body.*	mbali; mbail na katikati
distension *Swollen.*	uvimbe wa kibofu cha mkojo
distribution *The manner in which something is shared or spread out.*	usambazaji
diuresis *Increased excretion of urine.*	kuongeza uzalishaji wa mkojo
diuretic *Medication which causes an increased excretion of urine.*	kukojosha; dawa inayoongeza mkojo
dizziness *Sensation of losing one's balance.*	kizunguzungu; gumbizi
dorsal *Referring to the back or back surface.*	sehemu ya nyuma
dorsalis pedis pulse *Pulse on dorsum of the foot.*	juu ya wayo (mguuni) pahali moyo husikika ukipigia
dosage *The amount and frequency a medication is given.*	kipimo cha dawa
dosing interval *The number of times per unit a medication is given.*	kipimo kipindi
double *Twice the size, quantity or strength.*	mara mbili

English	Swahili
douche *Cleansing of a canal; unless otherwise specified it refers to cleansing of the vaginal canal.*	kusafisha ndani ya uke na maji au dawa
down *In a lower position.*	chini
drastic *Having significant effect.*	kuporomoka
dream *The thoughts or images occurring during sleep.*	ndoto
dressing *The gauze applied to a wound.*	bendeji
dribble, to *To slowly, drip-by-drip, release urine for example.*	piga chenga
drill *Cylindrical metal tool uses for creating a hole in bone in surgery.*	kekee
drink, to *To imbibe.*	kunywa
drinking water *Water clean enough to ingest orally.*	maji ya kunywa
drop *A single bit of fluid as in a drop seen while giving IV fluids.*	tone
drop by drop *Expression meaning little by little.*	kidogo kidogo
drops per minute *Refers to iv fluid rate.*	matone kwa dakika
drown,to *The process of dying from submerging in and inhaling water.*	kufa maji
drowsiness *Sleepiness. (in swahili ndezi also means rat)*	ndezi
drug *A medication, sometimes with negative connotation.*	dawa
drug dependence *Addiction to a substance.*	utegemezi wa dawa
drug reaction *Typically refers to an adverse effect of medication.*	mbaya ya athari kutokana na kutumia dawa
drunk *Inebriated.*	ulevi
dry *Absence of moisture.*	kavu
dry cough *A cough without sputum production.*	kavu kikohozi
dual diagnosis *Term used to describe the presence of alcohol/ drug addiction associated with a psychiatric diagnosis such as depression.*	ulevi na dhiki
duodenum *The portion of the small bowel between the stomach and jejunum.*	kwanza ya sehemu ya utumbo mdogo
duplication *The process of duplicating something.*	kurudia
dura mater *The outermost covering of the brain and spinal cord.*	upande wa nje wa ngozi ifunikayo ubongo na uti wa mgongo
dust *Dry earthen particles found on the ground and surfaces.*	vumbi
dwarf *Abnormally small person.*	kibeti; kibushuti
dysarthria *Difficulty in articulation of speech.*	ugumu akizungumza
dyschezia *Pain experienced during defecation.*	maumivu cha enda choo
dysentery *A severe form of diarrhea with blood and mucous in the stool.*	tumbo la kuhara
dyshidrosis *Disregulation of sweating*	usiokuwa wa kawaida jasho
dyskinesia *Abnormal movement.*	usiokuwa wa kawaida misuli harakati
dysmenorrhea *Pain during menstruation.*	maumivu ya hedhi
dyspepsia *Indigestion.*	kiungulia
dysphagia *Difficulty in swallowing.*	shida kumeza
dysphasia *Difficulty in speaking caused by cerebral dysfunction.*	ugumu akizungumza
dyspnea *Difficult breathing.*	kupumua kwa shida

71

English	Swahili
dysuria *Difficulty or pain upon urination.*	ugumu au maumivu na kukojoa
ear *The organ of hearing and balance.*	sikio
ear infection *General term referring to otitis media or otitis externa.*	sikio maambukizi
ear, inner *Auris interna.*	sikio la ndani
ear, middle *Auris media.*	katikati ya sikio
ear-drum *Common term for tympanic membrane.*	kiwambo cha sikio
earache *Pain associated with the ear.*	maumivu ya sikio
earlobe *The soft, fleshy inferior portion of the pinna.*	ndewe
eat, to *To consume food.*	kula
eating disorder *General term for pathologic eating habits.*	usiokuwa wa kawaida tabia ya kula
ecchymosis *Skin discoloration caused by bleeding beneath the epidermis.*	vilio la damu ngozini
eclampsia *A maternal condition characterized by convulsions and hypertension that can lead to maternal and fetal death.*	kifafa na shinikizo la damu wakati wa ujauzito
ectopic pregnancy *A pregnancy that is not intrauterine.*	mimba iliyo nje ya mji wake
ectropion *Eversion of the eyelid, usually the lower lid.*	ukope kuugeukia
eczema *A medical condition exhibited by pruritic, red, scaly patches on the scalp, cheeks and extensor surfaces.*	ukurutu
edema *Extravascular fluid accumulation.*	mapafu
education *Instruction or guidance.*	elimu
efficacious *Effective.*	ufanisi
effort *Attempt or endeavor.*	juhudi
ejaculation *The emission of semen at the moment of sexual climax in a male.*	kufukuza shahawa
elbow *The joint between the humerus and radius/ulna.(right elbow, left elbow)*	kisugudi
elderly *Advanced in years.*	wazee
elective *Non-urgent and not life-saving.*	hiari
elephantiasis *A condition caused by nematode parasites leading to lymphatic obstruction and limb or scrotal swelling.*	matende
elephantiasis of the scrotum *A condition caused by nematode parasites leading to lymphatic obstruction scrotal swelling.*	busha
elixir *A medical solution.*	dawa kufutwa katika kioevu
emaciation *Abnormally thin and weak.*	hali isiyo ya kawaida nyembamba na dhaifu
embolectomy *The removal of an embolus.*	kuondolewa kwa pande la damu
embolus *A blood clot, air bubble or fatty deposit that cause obstruction of a vessel.*	kuzibwa kwa mfereji wa damu na kidonge cha damu iliyoshikana
embryo *The term used to describe a fertilized ovum in the first 8 weeks of development.*	kiinitete
emergence *Coming into prominence.*	kuibuka
emergency *An urgent, life-threatening situation.*	dharura
emergency room *A ward used for initial treatment of critical patients.*	dharura chumba
emesis basin *A small bowl used to catch vomitus.*	ndogo bakuli kutumika kushikilia matapishi

English	Swahili
emesis *Vomit (noun)*	matapisha
emollient *Having softening or soothing qualities.*	dawa ya makuru kutumika kulainisha ngozi au kupunguza maumivu
emotion *An intense feeling.*	hisia
empathy *To be concerned for and share the feelings of another.*	uelewa
emphysema *Abnormal enlargement of the airspaces distal to the terminal bronchioles.*	kusakama kwa hewa mapafuni
empty *Containing nothing.*	tupu
empyema *A collection of purulent material in a body cavity, usually referring to a thoracic empyema.*	usaha katika mvungu wa mwili, kawaida kifua
encephalitis *Inflammation of the brain.*	kiwasho ya ugongo
encephalomyelitis *Inflammation of the brain and spinal cord.*	kiwasho wa ubongo na uti wa mgongo
encopresis *Involuntary defecation.*	si kukusudia haja kubwa
end point *The last stage of a process.*	mwisho kumweka
end stage *Terminal stage. End stage cancer means there is no cure possible and death is imminent.*	karibu na mwisho
endemic *When a disease is commonly found in a location or in a people group.*	wakati ugonjwa ni kupatikana kwa kawaida katika idadi ya watu
endometrium *The mucous membrane lining of the uterus.*	ukuta wa chungu cha mtoto
endotracheal *Within the trachea.*	within the umio wa pumzi
endow, to *To supply or provide for.*	kuyapatia
enema *A procedure involving insertion of fluid into the rectum.*	uwekaji wa maji katika mjiko
enlargement *Becoming bigger.*	utvidgningen
enormous *Very large.*	kubwa sana
ensure, to *To make certain of.*	kuhakikisha
ENT *Abbreviation for ears, nose and throat.*	masikio, pua na koo
enteral feeding *Nutrition supplied via the alimentary canal.*	kulisha ndani ya utumbo mdogo
enterectomy *Surgical resection of part of the intestine.*	upasuaji kuondoa sehemu ya utumbo mdogo
enteritis *Inflammation of the intestines.*	kiwasho ya utumbo mdogo
enucleation *Surgical removal of a globe.*	upasuaji kuondolewa kwa jicho
enuresis *Involuntary urination.*	si kukusudia kukojoa
enzyme *A compound that acts as a catalyst for reactions within cells as assists with digestion outside of cells.*	kimeng'enya
eosinophil *A cell with eosin stain used to designate a type of leukocyte that is elevated during allergic reactions.*	losinofili
epidemic *Ubiquitous development of an infectious disease.*	mlipuko
epidemiology *The study of the incidence, development and control of disease.*	magonjwa ya mlipuko
epidermis *The skin cells overlying the dermis.*	ngozi ya nje
epididymitis *Inflammation of the duct that moves sperm from the testis to the vas deferens.*	kufura kwa kiungo kalichoko nyuma ya kende
epidural *The space around the dura of the spinal cord.*	upande wa juu wa ngozi ifunikayo ubongona uti wa mgongo

73

English	Swahili
epigastrium *The section of the abdomen that overlies the stomach.*	tumbo, upande wa juu
epiglottis *Tissue at the base of the tongue that covers the trachea when one swallows.*	kidaka tonge
epilepsy *A condition associated with abnormal brain activity and exhibited by sudden, recurrent convulsions, sensory disturbances and loss of consciousness.*	kifafa
epileptic seizure *A convulsion related to abnormal brain activity (as opposed to being precipitated by hypoglycemia.)*	kifafa mshtuko
epistaxis *Bleeding emanating from the nose.*	muhina; damu inapotoka kwenye pua
equal *The same or uniform.*	sawa
equilibrium *When opposing forces are in balance.*	msawazisho
equipment *Apparatus or instrument.*	zana
erosion *The gradual destruction of surface tissue.*	mmomonyoko wa tishu
error *Mistake or inaccuracy.*	kosa
eructation *Belch or burp.*	mbweu
erysipelas *An acute infection caused by Streptococcus pyogenes that causes fever along with swelling and inflammation. The infection frequently effects the face or one leg.*	erisipela
erythrocyte *Called a red blood cell, it transports oxygen and carbon dioxide to and from the tissues.*	seli nyekundu za damu
eschar *Dry, hard, dead tissue commonly seen with a chronic pressure ulcer or anthrax.*	kavu, ngumu, wafu tishu
esophagectomy *Surgical removal of the esophagus.*	upasuaji kuondolewa umio
esophagitis *Inflammation of the esophagus.*	kiwasho ya umio
esophagus *The muscular tube that connects the throat to the stomach.*	umio ; umio wa chakula
essential *Crucial or necessary.*	muhimu
eunuch *A man who has been castrated.*	towashi
eustachian tube *The muscular canal that connects the tympanic membrane with the pharynx*	mfereji unaounganisha sikio na koo
evacuation *The emptying of an organ of fluids or gas.*	uokoaji
evaluation *Assessment or evaluation.*	tathmini
eversion *To turn outward.*	kugeuka nje
every day *Each day.*	kila siku
every *Each or all possible.*	kila
every other day *On alternate days.*	kila siku nyingine
evident *Obvious.*	dhahiri
evisceration *The removal of bowels from the body.*	viungo vya ndani vya tumbo kama vinaonekana na kutokea nje baada ya kidonda wazi
exacerbation *Worsening of an existing problem.*	mbaya ya tatizo lililopo
examination *Assessment or evaluation.*	upimaji
exanthema *A rash that accompanies a disease or fever.*	ngozi dalili za ugonjwa
excess *Surplus or overabundance.*	ziada
excrement *Feces.*	kinyesi
exfoliation *The shedding of scales.*	kumwaga ngozi

English	Swahili
exhumation *To remove a dead body from a grave.*	kuondoa maiti kutoka kaburini
exomphalos *Umbilical hernia.*	kichanga ngiri
exophthalmos *Protrusion of one or both eyeballs.*	mbenuko wa jicho
exostosis *A bony prominence growing from the surface of a bone.*	kinundu kwenye mfupa
exotropia *A type of strabismus that is characterized by the eyes turned outward.*	nje kugeuka ya macho
expansion *Enlargement or increase in size.*	upanuzi
expect, to *To suppose or presume.*	kutarajia
expectoration *The presence of sputum that has been coughed out.*	makohoo
expiration date *The date when a medication should no longer be used.*	tarehe ya kumalizika muda
expiration *Exhaling.*	kushusha pumzi
expiratory *Referring to exhalation of air from the lungs.*	kupumuliwa
exploratory laparotomy *Abdominal surgery with the intent of examining the abdominal contents.*	uchunguzi upasuaji wa tumbo
expulsion *Evacuation or elimination.*	kufukuzwa
expulsion of placenta *Passage of the placenta out the cervix after childbirth.*	kondo kufukuzwa
extend, to *To expand or stretch out.*	kunyoshea
external *Outside of the body.*	nje
extremity *Refers to one arm or one leg.*	mkono au mguu
extubation *The removal of a tube that was in a body orifice.*	kuondolewa kwa bomba kutoka kitundu mwili
exudate *The fluid, cells, and debris found in the tissues or a cavity (like pleural space) during inflammation.*	rishai
eye discharge *Conjunctival discharge.*	utongo
eye drops *Liquid applied to eyes for various medical problems.*	jicho matone
eyebrow *Supercilium.*	unyushi
eyeglasses *Eye wear used for cosmetic or prescription purposes.*	miwani
eyelash *Each of the short hairs on the eyelid.*	nywele juu ya ukope
eyelid *Palpebra.*	ukope
face *Anterior aspect of the head from the forehead to the chin.*	uso
face presentation *Referring to the part of the body coming out of the cervix first during childbirth.*	hali ya mtoto kutangulia na uso anapozaliwa
faint *Weak and dizzy.*	dhaifu na kizunguzungu
fainting *The act of losing consciousness.*	zimia; zirai
fair *Equitable.*	haki
fallopian tubes *Either of a pair of long narrow ducts located in a female's abdominal cavity that transport the male sperm cells to the egg.*	mrija kuunganisha ovari ya mji wa mimba
family	familia
family planning *Birth control.*	uzazi wa mpango
fascia *The fibrous sheath enclosing a muscle or organ.*	kitu kama kitambaa chembamba kinachozingira misuli (nyama)
fasting *Absence of caloric intake for a specified period.*	kufunga

75

English	Swahili
fat *A greasy or oiling substance naturally occurring in the body.*	mafuta
fatal *Lethal.*	kufisha
fatigue *Tiredness and exhaustion.*	uchovu
favus *Tinea capitis caused by Trichopyton schoenleini.*	aina ya bato
fear *Fright or trepidation.*	hofu
febrile *Presence of an supraphysiologic temperature.*	homa
fecal impaction *The presence of hard excrement in the rectum that requires manual removal.*	msongano kwa kinyesi
feces *Excrement.*	kinyesi
feel better or get better *To have improved health symptomatically.*	pata nafuu; pona
feel, to *To perceive or discern.*	kujisikia
female *Feminine.*	mwanamke
feminine pad *Gauze specially designed to absorb menstrual flow.*	sodo; usafi kitambaa
femur *The long bone in the thigh.*	mfupa wa paja
fertility *The ability of a person to contribute to contraception.*	uwezo wa kuzaa
fester, to *To become infected.*	tunga usaha
fetal distress *Term used to describe an abnormal heart rate or rhythm in a fetus indicating the need for urgent childbirth.*	mtoto ambaye hajazaliwa dhiki
fetal movements *Sensations by the mother of fetal activity.*	mtoto ambaye hajazaliwa harakati
fetal position *Refers to how the fetus lies within the uterus.*	mtoto ambaye hajazaliwa nafasi ndani ya mfuko wa uzazi
fetus *Medical term for the infant prior to birth.*	mimba
fever *A temperature above the normal range.*	homa
fibrin *An insoluble protein formed when fibrinogen is acted upon by thrombin.*	proteni isaidiayo kufanyika kwa vigaga au vidonge
fibrosis *Connective tissue that is scarred and thickened after injury.*	adilifu
fibula *The smaller of two bones in the lower leg.*	mfupa ndogo katika mguu chini
filiform *Threadlike.*	kama uzi
fimbria *A slender projection at the end of the fallopian tube near the ovary.*	vitu vinavyokaa kama vidole vya mkono mwishoni mwa mfereji wa fallopian
finger *Any of the five digits on the hand.*	kidole cha mkono
fingernail *Thin horny plate over the dorsal aspect of the end of finger.*	ukucha wa kidole cha mkono
fingertip *Distal aspect of a finger.*	ncha ya kidole cha mkono
firm *Hard or unyielding.*	imara
first aid *The initial treatment after an injury.*	huduma ya kwanza
fissure *A general term for a cleft or deep groove. An anal fissure, for example, is a small ulcer adjacent to the anus.*	ufa; mpasuko
fist *When a person has their fingers clenched tightly to the palm.*	ngumi
fistula *An abnormal communication between two organs or an organ and the skin, as in rectovaginal fistula.*	nasuri
flaccid *Limp. A term applied to an extremity one cannot move actively.*	teketeke

English	Swahili
flail chest *The term used when one has multiple rib fractures causing a segment of the chest wall to move incongruently with the rest of the chest wall.*	wakati bavu mbili au zaidi zimevunjika katika sehemu mbili au zaidi na kuacha sehemu ya ubavu imeninginia
flare-up *A sudden worsening one's condition.*	ghafla mbaya
flask *A narrow-necked container.*	chupa
flat *Level or even; without bulges.*	gorofa
flatfoot *Common term for pes planus.*	gorofa-mguu
flatulence *The gas expulsed from the anus.*	riahi
flatus *Term for air that is expelled from the anus.*	shuzi
flea *A small wingless insect that feeds on blood of mammals.*	kiroboto
flex *To bend.*	kunja
flow *Movement in a continuous stream.*	mtiririko
fluid intake *The amount of oral consumption plus the amount of intravenous fluids administered.*	maji ya ulaji
fluke *Parasitic nematode worm; an example is Schistosoma.*	ruba la ini
flutter *Used to describe a cardiac rhythm disturbance, as in atrial flutter.*	papatika
foam *A mass of small bubbles in a liquid.*	povu
fontanelle or fontanel *The space between the bones in the skull that are separate at birth.*	utosi
food intake *Quantitative record of nutritional intake.*	ulaji wa chakula
food *Nutrition.*	chakula
food poisoning *Poisoning where the active agent is in the food.*	chakula sumu
foot (sole of the foot) *The lower extremity distal to the ankle.*	wayo
foot and mouth disease *A contagious viral disease exhibited by oral and digital vesicles.*	ugonjwa wa midomo na miguu
foramen *An opening in a bone.*	tundu katika mfupa
foramen magnum *The hole in the skull that the spinal cord passes through.*	mwanya mkubwa upande wa chini wa kichwa ambapo uti wa mgongo hupitia
forceps *A surgical instrument, commonly called tweezers.*	koleo; kitindeo
forearm *Segment of the arm from the elbow to wrist.*	kigasha
forehead *Section of the face from the hairline to the eyebrows.*	kikoma cha uso; kidundu
forensic *Referring to the scientific method of studying crime.*	kuchunguza mauaji
foreskin *Also called prepuce, the skin that naturally covers the glans but can be rolled back.*	govi; zunga
former *Prior.*	zamani
forwards *Towards the front.*	mbele
fossa *A shallow depression.*	mvungu
fracture *A broken bone.*	mvunjiko wa mfupa
fracture, comminuted *A broken bone where one segment overrides the other.*	mvunjiko ambapo, mfupa umepondwa au kuvunjika kabisa
fracture, greenstick *A spiral fracture.*	kuvunjika ambako hakupenyi mfupa kabisa
framboesia; yaws *An endemic tropical disease caused by Treponema pertenue.*	buba

77

English	Swahili
free *Lacking or absent.*	kukosa au hayupo
frequency *Rate of occurrence.*	mzunguko
friable *Easily reduced to powder.*	mumuyika
friction *Grating or rasping.*	msuguano
frog *A tailless amphibian that is short with long hind legs for jumping.*	chura
frontal *Referring to the anterior aspect, as in frontal lobe.*	upande wa mbele
frostbite *Local tissue destruction after exposure to cold.*	jamidi
froth at the mouth, to *To have a mass of saliva with small bubbles in it coming out of the mouth.*	povu kinywani
froth *Covered with a mass of small bubbles.*	povu
frozen *Past participle of to freeze. Freeze: turn a liquid into a solid.*	waliohifadhiwa
frozen shoulder *Common term for adhesive capsulitis.*	ngumu bega
fungus *A spore-producing organism that feeds on organic matter.*	ukungu
furuncle *A painful erythematous nodule with a central core.*	jipu
gag *Choke or retch.*	jisua
gait *The way one walks.*	mwendo
gallbladder *The organ adjacent to the liver that stores bile and secretes it into the duodenum.*	kibofu cha nyongo
gallop *An abnormal heart sound.*	shoti
gallstone *Calculus produced in the bile duct or gallbladder.*	kijiwe katika kibofu cha nyongo
gangrene *Tissue death from either impaired blood flow or an infection.*	maradhi ya mti
gaping *Wide open.*	pengo
gargle, to *To rinse one's mouth out and exhale through the liquid.*	kusukutua
gastrectomy *Complete or partial surgical resection of the stomach.*	upasuaji kuondolewa kwa tumbo
gastric *Referring to the stomach.*	kusafisha mfuko wa tumbo
gastritis *Inflammation of the stomach.*	kiwasho ya mfuko wa tumbo
gastrocnemius *A large muscle in the lower leg, responsible for ankle plantar flexion, that is attached to the distal femur and achilles tendon.*	misuli:nyama za upande wa nyuma wa miguu
gastroduodenal ulcer *A lesion in the mucosal lining of the stomach or duodenum.*	kidonda katika mfuko wa tumbo na chango
gastroenteritis *A bacterial or viral infection that leads to vomiting and diarrhea.*	kufura kwa matumbo
gastrostomy *A surgical creation of an opening in the stomach.*	upasuaji viumbe wa ufunguzi katika mfuko wa tumbo
gauze *A fabric used for dressing changes.*	shashi ya pamba
gaze *Steady, intent look.*	mtazamo
gene *A unit of heredity that is passed on from parent to child.*	jeni
general appearance *The overall look of a patient.*	ujumla kuonekana
general *Common or expected.*	ujumla
genital ambiguity *A disorder of sexual development in which the genitalia are not sufficiently developed to tell clearly if the person is male or female.*	utata jinsia kitambulisho

English	Swahili
genital herpes *A sexually transmitted infection caused by herpes simplex.*	malengelenge sehemu za siri
genital wart *The common term for Condylomata acuminata.*	viungo vya uzazi chunjua
genitalia *Genitals.*	viungo vya uzazi
genu valgum *A condition exhibited by the knees turning inward, commonly referred to as knock-knee.*	kigosho cha miguu; yangekuwa goti
genu varum *A condition exhibited by the knees turning outward, commonly referred to as bowleg.*	chege
geriatrics *The study of the health of old people.*	huduma ya matibabu ya wazee
germ *Microorganism.*	kijidudu
German measles *(rubella) A contagious viral infection.*	kijerumani surua
gestation *The development of a fetus from conception until birth.*	ujauzito
get up out of bed	ondoka kitandani
giant *Huge or massive.*	kubwa au mkubwa
giardiasis *A flagellate protozoa, Giardia lamblia, that causes diarrhea.*	kiini chenye vitu kama nyuzi kipatikanacho kwenye maji ya juu
giddiness *A tendency to fall or dizziness.*	kizunguzungu; masua
gingival *Referring to the gums.*	ufizi
gingivitis *Inflammation of the gums.*	kiwasho wa ufizi
glance *A brief look at something.*	mtazamo
glans penis *The distal aspect of the penis.*	akipiga sehemu ya uume; kichwa cha mboo
glare *An angry stare.*	kodoa macho
Glasgow coma scale *A scale used to grade one's level of consciousness with a score of 3 being totally unresponsive and a score of 15 being normal.*	glascow kukosa fahamu wadogo
glaucoma *A condition characterized by increased intraocular pressure.*	glakoma
glossectomy *Surgical resection of the whole or part of the tongue.*	upasuaji kuondolewa kwa ulimi
glossitis *Inflammation of the tongue.*	kiwasho wa ulimi
glossodynia *Tongue pain.*	maumivu wa ulimi
glottis *Essentially the vocal structure, including the true vocal cords and the opening between them.*	viungo vya kutoa sauti na nafasi iliyo kati kati ya viungo hivyo
gloves *Covering for hand protection.*	glavu
glucagon *A pancreatic enzyme responsible for breakdown of glycogen to glucose.*	kitu kinachochochea kuongezeka kwa sukari kwenye damu
glue *Plastic cements*	gundi
gluteal or gluteus muscle *A paired set of three muscles, the gluteus maximus, medius and minimus, that all have origins in the ilium and insertions in the femur. (buttocks)*	misuli nyama za matako
glycosuria *Presence of glucose in the urine.*	sukari katika mkojo
gnosia *Ability to recognize things and people.*	ukosefu wa uwezo wa kutambua mambo au watu
go to the doctor, to	kwenda kwa daktari
go to the hospital, to	kwenda hospitali

English	Swahili
goiter *Swelling of the thyroid gland.*	rovu; goita
gold *Precious metal with atomic number of 79.*	dhahabu
gonad *A testis or an ovary.*	koko au ovari
gonorrhea *A sexually transmitted disease that is exhibited by purulent discharge from the vagina or penis.*	kisonono
gonorrheal arthritis *A type of arthritis caused by the gram negative diplococcus Neisseria gonorrhoeae.*	ugua mifupa na kisonono
gonorrheal ophthalmia *An acute purulent conjunctivitis that can occur in neonates within 2-5 days of birth.*	kisonono jicho ugonjwa
goose bumps *Cutis anserina.*	kimbimbi
gout *Monosodium urate crystal deposition disease.*	jongo
gown *A sterile gown used during surgical procedures.*	upasuaji kanzu
graft *A piece of tissue surgically transplanted.*	pandikiza
Graves' disease *A form of hyperthyroidism exhibited by a goiter and exophthalmos.*	tezi na kororo
gravida *Pregnant.*	wajawazito
greater than normal *Above normal.*	kubwa kuliko kawaida
grief *Deep sorrow.*	huzuni
groan *A deep inarticulate sound made due to pain or despair.*	tunaugua
groin pull *A muscle strain in the inguinal region.*	kinena misuli kuumia
groin *The genital region.*	kinena ; manena
growth *The increase in physical size.*	endeleo
guarding *A symptom used to describe a patient resisting an examination because of severe pain; often seen in patients with peritonitis.*	kupinga mitihani kwa sababu ya maumivu
guinea worm *A parasitic nematode worm that, in cases of infection, lives under the skin, formally called Dracunculus medinensis.*	Guinea ya mdudu
gum *Gingiva.*	ufizi
gumboil *Swelling noted on the gingiva over a dental abscess.*	jipu kwenye ufizi
gumma *A soft granulomatous tumor of the skin or cardiovascular system seen in tertiary syphilis.*	mtoki dalili ya kaswende elimu ya juu
gunshot wound *An penetrating injury sustained from a bullet.*	risasi na jeraha
gustatory agnosia *The loss of the sense of taste.*	ukosefu wa maana ya ladha
gynecomastia *Enlargement of the breasts.*	utvidgningen ya matiti
habit *A custom or inclination.*	zoezi
hair (of body) {axillary and pubic hair}	mwili nywele; {vuzi}
hair (of head) {facial hair- beard}	nywele juu ya kichwa {udevu}
half *Divided in two.*	nusu
half-life *The time a drug decreases its effect in half over time.*	nusu ya maisha
halitosis *Foul odor emanating from the mouth.*	mbaya pumzi
hallucination *A perception that is not based on reality.*	wazimu; maruerue
hallux valgus *Also called bunion, it is the lateral deviation of the great toe.*	imara kupotoka ya gumba
hallux varus *Medial deviation of the great toe.*	ndani kupotoka ya gumba
hamstrings *Tendons of the posterior thigh.*	misuli nyama za mguu upande wa nyuma
hand *The upper extremity distal to the wrist.*	mkono

80

English	Swahili
hand, dorsum *Back of hand. (kingaja also means bracelet)*	kingaja
hand, left	mkono wa kushoto
hand, palm of	kitanga cha mkono; kiganja
hand, right	mkono wa kulia
hangnail *A loose piece of skin attached near the medial or lateral nail fold.*	kikuchia; kigozikucha
Hansen's disease *Leprosy*	ukoma

English-Swahili: hard of hearing-myelitis

English	Swahili
hard of hearing *Decreased sense of hearing.*	kupungua kusikia
hard *Rigid or very firm.*	ngumu
harmless *Safe or benign.*	wapole
hazy *Cloudy.*	machafu
head	kichwa
head trauma *Any injury to the brain.*	kuumia kwa ubongo
headache *Cephalgia.*	maumivu cha kichwa
healing *The process of becoming healthy again.*	uponyaji
health center *A physical location where patients are treated.*	kituo cha faya
health *The state of being free of illness.*	afya
healthy *In good health.*	nawiri
hearing aid *A device that fits in the ear used to amplify sound.*	kusikia misaada
hearing *Auditory perception.*	kusikia kwa masikio
heart beat *A single contraction of the heart.*	pigo la moyo
heart disease *Generic term generally meant to imply coronary disease.*	afkani
heart murmur *An abnormal heart sound usually related to valvular disease.*	moyo msinung'unike
heart *Muscular organ that pumps blood thru the circulatory system.*	moyo
heart rate *Number or cardiac contractions per minute.*	kwingo cha moyo
heartburn *Synonym of pyrosis.*	kiungulia
heat exhaustion *A condition that occurs secondary to prolonged exposure to high ambient temperature; it is exhibited by subnormal temperature, dizziness and nausea.*	udhaifu unaotokana na kupoteza maji kwa ajili ya kutokwa na jasho kupita kiasa
heat stroke *A condition caused by excessive exposure to high ambient temperature; it is exhibited by dry skin, thirst, vertigo, muscle cramps and nausea. The three forms are heat exhaustion, heat cramps and sunstroke.*	joto kiharusi
heat *The quality of being hot.*	joto
heavy *Possessing great weight.*	nzito
heel *Proximal portion of the plantar aspect of the foot.*	kisigino cha mguu
heel-shin test (heel to knee to toe test) *A test of position sense and coordination; one moves the heel of one foot from the knee on the other foot down to the foot.*	kisigino cha mguu-muundi mtihani
height *Distance between the bottom of the foot and top of the head.*	kimo cha mtu
hematemesis *Vomiting blood.*	kutapika damu
hematochezia *Presence of blood in the excrement.*	umwagaji damu kinyesi
hematoma *A mass containing blood.*	damu inapojikusanya pamoja
hematuria *The presence of blood in the urine.*	kojoa damu
hemeralopia *Night blindness.*	upofu wa usiku

82

English	Swahili
hemiparesis *Unilateral muscle weakness (half the body).*	udaifu unaoathiri upande mmoja wa mwili
hemiplegia *Paralysis of one side of the body.*	ulemavu wa mwili nusu
hemoglobin *An iron containing protein used for the transport of oxygen in blood.*	rangi nyekundu ya damu
hemolysis *Breakdown of hemoglobin.*	kuvunjika kwa rangi nyekundu ya damu
hemopericardium *Abnormal presence of blood in the pericardium.*	usiokuwa wa kawaida uwepo wa damu kuzunguka bitana ya moyo
hemophilia *A hereditary bleeding disorder characterized by hemarthroses and deep tissue bleeding as a result of absence of a coagulation factor such as factor VIII.*	kurithi damu machafuko
hemophthalmia *Bleeding within the eye.*	kutokwa na damu ndani ya jicho
hemopoiesis *The production of blood cells from stem cells.*	kufanyizwa kwa damu
hemoptysis *Expectoration of blood.*	kukohoa damu
hemorrhage *Bleeding from a damaged blood vessel.*	kuvuja kwa damu
hemorrhoidectomy *Surgical excision of a hemorrhoid.*	upasuaji kuondolewa kwa bawasiri
hemorrhoids *Engorgement of the veins in the anus or rectum.*	bawasiri
hemostasis *The control of bleeding.*	udhibiti wa damu
hemothorax *The abnormal presence of blood in the pleural cavity.*	usiokuwa wa kawaida uwepo wa damu katika kifua
hence *Thus.*	hivyo
hepatectomy *Partial or complete surgical resection of the liver.*	upasuaji kuondolewa kwa ini
hepatitis *Inflammation of the liver.*	kiwasho cha ini
hepatomegaly *Enlargement of the liver.*	upanuzi wa ini
hereditary *That which is transmitted genetically*	kurithiwa
hermaphrodite *A person possessing gonadal characteristics of both sexes.*	huntha
hernia *An abnormal bulge of bowel through muscle.*	ngiri
hernia, inguinal *Protrusion of abdominal-cavity contents through the inguinal canal.*	kinena ngiri
hernia, umbilical *Protrusion of abdominal contents at the umbilicus.*	kichanga ngiri
herniorrhaphy *The surgical repair of a hernia.*	upasuaji wa ngiri kukarabati
herpes *A skin condition exhibited by formation of clustered vesicular lesions; herpes simplex is at times referred to, albeit incompletely, as herpes.*	malengelenge; manawa
herpes zoster; shingles *A unilateral vesicular rash along one dermatome and caused by inflammation of a posterior nerve root by "the chicken pox virus".*	mkanda wa jeshi
heterogenous *That which originates outside the organism.*	kumba
hiccup *Involuntary spasm of the diaphragm with sudden closure of the glottis; this causes a characteristic cough.*	kwikwi; chechevu
hidradenitis *Inflammation of a sweat gland. When there is purulent discharge it is called hidradenitis suppurativa.*	kiwasho cha jasho tezi
high altitude cerebral edema	ugonjwa wa akilini kutokana na kupanda juu mlimani

high altitude pulmonary edema — kufura kwa mapafu kutokana na kuwa juu sana

high blood pressure *Elevated arterial blood pressure.* — shinikizo la damu

high *Elevated.* — juu

hip *The lateral eminence of the pelvis from the waist to the thigh; it is formed by the iliac crest and greater trochanter.* — nyonga

hip replacement *Both joint surfaces are replaced by high density material such as plastic or metal.* — upasuaji badala ya nyonga

hirsutism *Abnormal growth on hair on a person's face and body.* — nywele kuruwili

histamine *A chemical responsible for the reaction exhibited when a person has an allergic reaction.* — kitu cha kiasili kwenye mwili kinachopigana na majeraha au na kitu chochoke kigeni mwilini

histoplasmosis *A fungal pulmonary infection from bat and bird excrement.* — vimelea mapafu maambukizi yanayosababishwa na kinyesi ndege

HIV *Abbreviation for human immunodeficiency virus.* — vijidudu virusi

hives *Urticaria* — ugonjwa wa mabaka ngozini

hoarse *A rough, harsh sounding voice.* — uchakacho

hollow *An indentation.* — uvungu

homicide *When one person kills another.* — kuua mwingine

hookworm *A parasitic infection of the family Strongylidae that can cause anemia.* — kidusia vinavyosababisha maambukizi ya upungufu wa damu

hordeolum *Inflammation of the sebaceous gland of the eye.* — chokea

hospital *Acute care medical/surgical facility.* — hospitali

hospital discharge *To leave the hospital.* — kuondoka hospitali

hot *Very warm.* — moto

human *Homo sapien.* — binadamu

humerus *The long bone in the upper arm.* — mfupa wa mkono katikati ya kiko na bega

hunchback *Synonym of kyphosis.* — kigongo

hunger *A sense of discomfort caused by a lack of food.* — njaaa

hydration *Used to describe fluid balance.* — taratibu

hydrocele *The accumulation of fluid in a body sac.* — kiboleini

hydrocephalus *The excessive accumulation of cerebral spinal fluid in the brain causing enlargement of the head.* — mkusanyiko wa maji katika ubongo

hydrophobia *Abnormal fear of water.* — usiokuwa wa kawaida hofu ya maji

hydrothorax *Accumulation of fluid within the thoracic cavity.* — usiokuwa wa kawaida mkusanyiko wa maji katika kifua

hymen *A membrane in the vagina.* — kizinda

hyperbaric *Use of gas at a higher than normal pressure.* — yenye nguvu; uzito mwingi

hyperglycemia *Higher than normal level of glucose in the blood.* — iliongezeka sukari katika damu

hyperhidrosis *Excessive perspiration.* — kupindukia jasho

hypermnesia *Unusually good memory.* — isiyo ya kawaida na kumbukumbu nzuri

English	Swahili
hyperopia *Farsightedness.*	uwezo wa kuona katika umbali mkubwa
hyperphagia *Excessive food ingestion.*	kupindukia chakula kumeza
hyperpigmentation, skin disease causing *General term to describe skin darkening.*	mbulanga
hyperpnea *Abnormal increase in rate and depth of respiration.*	kuongezeka kwa kiwango na kina cha kupumua
hyperpyrexia *Fever.*	homa
hypersensitivity *Abnormal increase in sensitivity.*	usiokuwa wa kawaida kuongezeka kwa unyeti
hypertension *Higher than normal blood pressure.*	shinikizadamu
hyperthermia *Fever.*	homa
hypertrichosis *Excessive hair growth.*	nywele nyingi ukuaji
hyperventilation *Rapid and deep respirations.*	kupumua haraka bila sababu
hypnotic *Sleep inducing agent.*	madawa ambayo husababisha usingizi
hypoesthesia *Abnormally decreased skin sensitivity.*	ilipungua ngozi unyeti
hypogastrium *The area of the central abdomen located below the stomach.*	kinena
hypoglycemia *Abnormally low blood sugar.*	hali ya kupungua kwa sukari kwenye damu
hypotension *Abnormally low blood pressure.*	chini ya shinikizo la damu
hypothalamus *Located inferior to the thalamus it controls visceral activities, water balance, temperature and sleep.*	sehemu ya ubongo ambayo huzimamia baadhi ya kazi za mwili kama urekebishaji wa joto
hypothermia *Lower than normal temperature.*	hali isiyo ya kawaida chini joto la mwili
hypoxia *Diminished oxygen content.*	kuwa na kiasi kidogo cha hewa ya oxygen
hysterectomy *Surgical removal of the uterus.*	upasuaji kuondolewa kwa mfuko wa uzazi
hysteria *A psychological condition exhibited by uncontrolled emotion or exaggerated manifestations.*	kupugawa
iatrogenic *A problem caused by medical treatment.*	tatizo unasababishwa na matibabu
ichthyosis *A congenital anomaly exhibited by excessively dry, thick skin.*	kuzaliwa abnormality: kupita kiasi kavu ngozi
icterus *Yellowing of the skin and sclerae because of excess bilirubin.*	homa ya manjano
identical twins *Twins from the same zygote.*	kufanana mapacha
idiopathic *Relating to a disease with an unknown cause.*	sababu haijulikani
ilium *The large bone at the superior aspect of the pelvis which is present bilaterally.*	tokoni
illiterate *Unable to read or write.*	hawajui kusoma na kuandika
immersion foot *After prolonged cold exposure the foot is cold and numb. As it rewarms, it becomes hyperemic, paresthetic and hyperhidrotic.*	jeraha la baridi ambalo sio la kuganda ambalo huletwa na baridi au majimaji hali inayozuia damu kutembea vizuri

85

English	Swahili
immune *Being resistant to an infection.*	kingamwili
immunization *A medication given to provide immunity.*	chanjo
immunodeficiency *An inadequate immune response.*	ukosefu wa kinga mwilini
impaction, tooth *A tooth that does not erupt because adjacent teeth prevent it.*	meno msongano
impairment *A specific disability.*	kuharibika
imperforate *Lack of an opening. An infant with an imperforate anus has a congenital defect with no anal opening.*	ukosefu wa ufunguzi
impervious *Not affected by.*	huweza kuingia
impetigo	upele wa malengelenge
implementation *The process of putting a plan into effect.*	utekelezaji
impotence *Inability to act or inability to achieve a penile erection.*	mkuwadi
inarticulate *Indistinct speech.*	si wazi hotuba
incision *An intentional surgical cut in the skin.*	chale
incisor *Sharp-edged tooth; humans have four incisors.*	jino la mbele
incoherent *Absence of intelligible speech.*	ukosefu wa hotuba ya kueleweka
incontinence *Inability to control urination.*	kukosa uwezo wa kudhibiti kukojoa
incoordination *Absence of smooth, efficient body movement.*	Kukosa mwelekeo
increment *An increase on a fixed scale.*	Unaozidi
incubator *A warming device for infants.*	kitanda zimefungwa kifaa cha joto
indeed *As a matter of fact.*	kweli
indigenous *Naturally occurring.*	kiasili
indolent *1. Causing little pain. 2. Slow healing ulcer.*	goigoi
induce, to *Facilitated. When referring to labor, it means medication was given to assist in delivery of the fetus.*	kushawishi
induced abortion *Surgical or medical evacuation of the fetus.*	ikiwa utoaji mimba
induration *An area that is abnormally hard.*	gumu
indwelling catheter *Continuous use tube usually referring to a tube in the urinary bladder.*	kasiba ya kukaa katika kibofu cha mkojo mkojo
inebriation *Intoxication with drugs or alcohol.*	nishai
ineffective *Unsuccessful or inefficient.*	ufanisi
inertia *The tendency to remain unchanged.*	hali
inevitable *Not preventable.*	kuepukika
infancy *Early childhood.*	uchanga
infant *Newborn.*	watoto wachanga
infarct *Referring to dead tissue.*	akimaanisha tishu wafu
infectious *Contagious.*	kuambukiza
infectious disease *Any disease or condition considered contagious.*	ugonjwa wa kuambukiza
inferior *The lower aspect.*	chini nyanja
inflammation *Localized redness, excessive warmth and swelling.*	kiwasho
influenza *Viral infection causing fever, muscle aches and catarrh. (bombo also means pair of shorts in swahili)*	bombo

English	Swahili
infusion *The injection of fluid into tissue or a vein.*	sindano ya maji katika mshipa
ingestion *The intake of food or liquid orally.*	kumeza
ingrown nail *Also referred to as onychocryptosis.*	kiwasho ngozi karibu ukucha
inguinal *Referring to the groin.*	kinena
inhalation *The act of breathing in.*	kuvuta pumzi
injection *The act of a needle being inserted into a body. (given injection)*	sindano (choma sindano)
injure, to *To hurt or to wound.*	kuwadhuru
injury *A wound, abrasion or contusion.*	kuumia ; dhara; jeraha
inoculation *Injection with a vaccine to provide immunity.*	chanjo
insane *A term not used in formal medical evaluations that when used by a layperson means a serious mental illness.*	mwendawazimu
insanity *Referring to a serious mental illness.*	kichaa; wazimu
insect bite	umo la mdudu ngozini
insertion *The act of inserting something.*	kuingizwa
inside *Inner part, center.*	ndani ya
insidious *A slow, gradual and harmful advancement.*	polepole, taratibu mwanzo
insomnia *Sleeplessness.*	usingizi
inspiration *Drawing in a breath.*	kuvuta pumzi
instep *The medial aspect of the foot between the ankle and the ball of the foot.*	mvungo wa wayo
insulin *A hormone produced by the pancreas and synthetically to control blood glucose levels.*	dawa ambayo hupunguza viwango vya sukari damu
intensive care *Vigorous treatment of the acutely ill.*	wagonjwa mahututi
intention tremor *The tremulous movement noted when a person is beginning to perform a task but not seen at rest.*	tetemeko alibainisha wakati wa harakati, si katika mapumziko
intercostal *Area between the ribs*	katikati ya mbavu
intermittent *Occurring at irregular intervals.*	vipindi
internal *Situated on the inside.*	ndani ya
interval *An intervening time.*	muda
intestinal obstruction *Blockage of the intestine by mass or volvulus.*	matumbo kizuizi
intestine *A general term used for the section of bowel from the stomach to the anus.*	matumbo
intraabdominal abscess *A collection of pus in the abdomen.*	ndani ya tumbo jipu
intraabdominal *Within the abdominal cavity.*	ndani ya tumbo
intracerebral *Within the cerebrum.*	ndani ya ubongo
intracranial *Within the cranial vault.*	ndani ya fuvu
intramuscular *Within a muscle.*	ndani ya misuli
intraosseous *Within a bone.*	ndani ya mfupa
intrauterine contraceptive device (IUD) *A device used to physically prevent the implantation of a fertilized ovum.*	mibinu for kuzuia mimba ndani ya mfuko la uzazi
intrauterine *Within the uterus.*	ndani ya mfuko la uzazi
intravenous *Within a vein.*	kupitia kwa mishipa ya vena
inversion *Turning inward.*	kuingia kwa ndani
involuntary movement *Movement not controlled consciously.*	mwendo usio wa hiari

English	Swahili
iodine *A chemical used as an antiseptic and a deficiency of it can lead to goiter.*	madini
ipsilateral *On the same side.*	upando huo
iron *An element found in hemoglobin.*	feri
iron-deficiency anemia *A microcytic anemia.*	feri upungufu safura
irrelevant *Not pertinent.*	lisilo
ischemia *Inadequate blood supply to a part of the body.*	haitoshi damu ugavi
ischium *The inferoposterior portion of the pelvis.*	mfupa wa kitako
isolation ward *A ward where patients with infectious disease are housed.*	kutengwa eneo
itch *A sensation that makes one want to scratch.*	ukuruti
jaundice of the newborn *A form of jaundice seen in newborns in the first two weeks of life; also called icterus neonatorum.*	homa ya manjano ya mtoto mchanga
jaundice *Yellowing of the sclerae and skin because of excessive bilirubin in the blood.*	homa ya manjano
jaw *Mandible.*	taya
jock itch *Pruritus caused by tinea cruris.*	choa ya kinena
joint *Articulation of two adjacent bones.*	kiungo (viungo)
jugular vein (s) *Includes the internal, external and anterior jugular veins.*	damu chombo kwamba anarudi damu kutoka kwenye ubongo na moyo
jugular venous distension *Enlarged jugular veins caused by high pulmonary capillary pressure.*	hali ambapo vena ya shingo hupanuka
juxta-articular *Positioned near a joint.*	karibu na kiungo
kala-azar *A disease caused by Leishmania donovani that is exhibited by weight loss, fever, anemia and hepatosplenomegaly.*	ugonjwa wa sarufa, homa na upanuzi wengu unasababishwa na Leishmenia
Kaposi sarcoma *Typically seen in AIDS patients, it is characterized by cutaneous reddish-purple macules and plaques. Also called multiple idiopathic hemorrhagic sarcoma.*	Kaposis sarcoma
keloid *Hypertrophic scar tissue that forms after a minor cut or surgical procedure.*	kova tishu
keratin *A protein found in the skin, hair, nails and enamel of the teeth.*	proteni ngumu kwenye ngozi, kucha na nywele
kick, to *To strike an object with one's foot.*	kupiga teke
kidney *One of two glandular organs that form urine.*	figo; buki
knee *The joint at the distal femur and proximal tibia.*	goti
knee elbow position *Knees and elbows are on the table and the chest is in the air.*	fuama
kneecap *Common term for patella.*	pia ya mguu; kilegesambwa
kneeling *Being on one's knees as in the prayer position.*	pia magoti
knock knees *Common term for genu valgum.*	kigosho cha miguu; yangekuwa goti
knot *A fastening made by tying a suture, for instance.*	fundo
known *Recognized or familiar.*	inayojulikana
knuckles *Metacarpophalangeal joints or finger joints when the fist is closed.*	nguyu
koilonychia *Thin and concave fingernails.*	nyembemba na vungu ukucha wa kidole cha mkono;

English	Swahili
kwashiorkor *A form of malnutrition from inadequate protein intake.*	utapio mlo
kyphosis *Abnormal outward curvature of the spine.*	kigongo
lab result *The data obtained from a laboratory test.*	maabara ya matokeo
labium *Referring to any lip shaped structure.*	mdomo
labor onset *The time when a pregnant woman begins uterine contractions in the process of childbirth.*	mwanzo wa kuzaa; pata uchungu wa kuzaa
labor pains *The intermittent pain associated with uterine contractions.*	uchungu wa kuzaa
laboratory test	uchunguzi wa maabara
lacrimal fluid *Fluid secreted by the lacrimal gland.*	machozi
lacrimal *Referring to the secretion of tears.*	inao uhusiano na machozi
lacrimation *The secretion of tears.*	uzalishaji ya machozi
lactation *The secretion of milk from mammary glands.*	utoaji wa maziwa
lagophthalmos *Characterized by the inability to close the eyelid completely over the eye.*	kutokuwa na uwezo wa kuifunga (nywele juu) ya ukope juu ya jicho
lancet *A small sharp instrument used to obtain a drop of blood for testing.*	kijembe
laparotomy *A surgical incision of the abdomen.*	upasuaji wa tumbo chale
laryngectomy *Surgical removal of the larynx.*	upasuaji kuondolewa ya zoloto
laryngitis *Inflammation of the larynx.*	kiwasho ya zoloto
laryngospasm *Sudden, involuntary muscle contraction of the larynx.*	si kwa hiari misuli kipindupindu ya zoloto
laryngotomy *Surgical creation of an opening in the larynx.*	upasuaji viumbe wa ufunguzi katika zoloto
larynx *A hollow muscular structure that contains the vocal cords.*	zoloto; kikoromeo
last *Final.*	mwisho
late *A time later than expected.*	chelewa
lateral *Referring to the side of the body.*	upande
laugh, to	kucheka
laxity *A description of a joint that is loose. (ndezi also means rat in Swahili)*	ndezi
layer *A stratum or thickness.*	tabaka
lead *An element with an atomic number of 82.*	tindikali
lead poisoning *The ingestion of lead, exhibited in severe cases by paralysis, encephalopathy, purple gingiva, and colic.*	sumu tindikali (plumbi)
leakage *Unintentional escape of gas or fluid.*	kuvuja
learning *The intentional acquisition of knowledge.*	kujifunza
leech *An annelid used in some tropical regions for drawing out blood; they have an anticoagulant effect locally and have been attached to digits of persons with acute peripheral ischemia.*	mruba
left	kushoto
left-handed *The preference of using the left hand for common tasks.*	shoto
leg *One of two lower extremities.*	mguu

English	Swahili
leishmaniasis *A condition caused by a flagellate protozoan parasite that is exhibited by visceral or dermatologic manifestations.*	ugonjwa wa sarufa, homa na upanuzi wengu unasababishwa na Leishmenia
length *The end to end measurement.*	urefu
lengthening *Becoming longer.*	kurefusha
lens *The transparent chamber between the posterior chamber and the vitreous body.*	lenzi
leprosy *A contagious disease caused by Mycobacterium leprae that causes insensate papules and disfiguration.*	ukoma
less *A smaller amount.*	chini ya
lethal *Deadly.*	mauti
lethal dose *The amount of a drug required to cause death.*	mauti dosi
lethargy *Absence of energy.*	uchovu
leukocyte *A white blood cell.*	seli nyeupe ya damu
leukorrhea *Thick white vaginal discharge.*	nene nyeupe ukeni
lice *Plural for louse, a small parasite that lives on the skin. Pediculus humanus capitis is a head louse.*	chawa
life expectancy *The length of time a person is anticipated to live.*	urefu wa muda mtu anatarajiwa kuishi
life-threatening *Potentially fatal.*	kutishia maisha
lifetime *Duration of a person's life.*	maisha
lift, to *Raise to a higher level.*	kuinua
ligament *A band of fibrous connective tissue that connects two bones or cartilage.*	nyama nyembamba kama mshipa inayounganisha mfupa kwa mwingine
ligature *A thread used to tie a vessel.*	mshono kutumika kufunga chombo damu
light *Illumination, bright.*	nuru
light *Not heavy.*	epesi
likelihood *The probability or feasibility.*	uwezekano
lip, lower *Labium inferius oris.*	chini mdomo
lip, upper *Labium superius oris.*	juu mdomo
lipoma *A benign tumor consisting of fat cells.*	mafuta donge
lisping *A speech problem in which "s" and "z" are pronounced "th".*	kusema kitembe
liver *A large glandular organ in the right upper quadrant that functions in digestive processes, as well as, neutralizing toxins.*	ini
liver abscess *A localized collection of pus in the liver.*	ini jipu
localized *Toward one point or area.*	kuelekea hatua moja au eneo
loculated *Divided into small cavities.*	kugawanywa katika mashimo madogo
long-acting *Referring to a drug with long lasting effects.*	muda kaimu
long-standing *Having existed for a long time.*	muda mrefu
longevity *Long life.*	maisha marefu
longsighted *Synonym of hyperopia.*	muda mrefu wenye kuona
loose *Not tight.*	kulegea
loss of consciousness *Unresponsive to verbal and tactile stimuli.*	kupoteza fahamu
lots of *An abundance of.*	kura ya

90

English	Swahili
low back pain *Pain in the lumbar region.*	chini kiuno maumivu
lower extremity edema *Interstitial edema of the legs.*	mguu wa mapafu
lubricant *Emollient.*	lainisha kwa mafuta
lumbago *Pain in the region of the lumbar spine.*	chini kiuno maumivu
lumbar *Referring to the spinal region inferior to the thoracic spine.*	kiuno
lump *A protuberance.*	pande; rugurugu
lung *One of a pair of respiratory organs.*	pafu
lymph *A transparent and sometimes opalescent fluid that flows in the lymph channels.*	limfu
lymph node *An area of organized lymphatic tissue.*	limfu nodi
lymphangitis *Inflammation of the lymph vessels.*	kuvimba kwa mefereji na vyombo vya maji ya mwilini
lymphocyte *A white blood cell produced by the lymph tissue.*	limfosaiti
lymphoma *A malignant disease of the lymph system, Hodgkin's lymphoma for example.*	limfu, aina nyingi
macrocheilia *Abnormally large lips.*	hali isiyo ya kawaida kubwa midomo
macrodactyly *Abnormally large digits.*	hali isiyo ya kawaida kubwa vidole
macroencephaly *Having an abnormally large head.*	hali isiyo ya kawaida kubwa kichwa
macroglossia *Abnormally large tongue.*	hali isiyo ya kawaida kubwa ulimi
macula solaris *Formal medical term describing a freckle.*	doa ngozini
mad cow disease *Bovine spongiform encephalopathy, a disease that cause cerebral degeneration exhibited by ataxia.*	ng'ombe wazimu ugonjwa
madness *Common term for insanity.*	wazimu; kichaa
magnet *A piece of iron with atoms ordered to make it magnetic.*	sumaku
malaise *A vague feeling of discomfort or unease.*	uchovu; kujisikia vibaya
malaria *A condition caused by a protozoan of the genus Plasmodium. It is transmitted by mosquitos and is exhibited by fever, chills, headache. In the severe form it can lead to convulsions, increased ICP and death.*	homa ya mbu; malaria
malignant *Tendency of a tumor to invade normal tissue.*	hatari
malingerer *A person who feigns illness.*	kujifanya kuwa wagonjwa
malleolus *A bony protrusion on medial and lateral aspect of each ankle.*	mwishoni mwa mufupa miwili ya miguuni pahali imechukua muundo wa muiringo
malnutrition *Lack of appropriate nutrition.*	utapiamlo
mammary *Referring to the breast.*	akimaanisha matiti
man *Male human.*	mwanamume
management *The process of dealing with things or people.*	usimamizi
mandatory *Obligatory.*	lazima
mandible *The lower jaw.*	taya la chini
mania *A mental disorder exhibited by hyperexcitability, delusions and euphoria.*	mahoka
marasmus *Progressive weight loss and emaciation.*	maendeleo ya kupoteza uzito
marijuana *Cannabis.*	bangi

English	Swahili
marital counseling *Therapy aimed at marriage reconciliation.*	ndoa ushauri nasaha
marital status *Single versus married status.*	hadhi ya ndoa
marsupialization *Creation of a surgical pouch.*	kuundwa kwa kifuko ya upasuaji
mass *Tumor.*	kitonge
mastectomy *Surgical resection of one or both breasts.*	upasuaji kuondolewa moja au zote mbili matiti
mastication *Chewing.*	kutafuna
mastitis *Inflammation of the breast.*	kiwasho cha matiti
mastodynia *Breast pain.*	maumivu cha matiti
mastoid *Referring to the mastoid process.*	nyuma sehemu ya mfupa kidunia
matching *Corresponding in pattern or style.*	vinavyolingana
mattress *A fabric case filled with material, used for sleeping.*	magodoro
maxilla *The upper jaw that also forms the inferior portion of the orbit and part of the nose.*	kituguta
meaningless *Having no significance.*	maana
measles *A childhood viral, infectious disease exhibited by rash and fever.*	surua; ukambi
meconium *The first newborn feces which are green.*	kwanza waliozaliwa kinyesi kuchanganywa na maji yanayozunguka kijusi
medial *Situated toward the midline.*	katikati ; karibu na katikati
mediastinum *The thoracic area between the lungs.*	eneo la kifua kati ya mapafu
medication *A substance used for medical treatment.*	tembe; dawa; vidonge
medicine *A substance used for medical treatment or the art and science of healing patients.*	tembe; dawa; vidonge
medicine, to get	kupata dawa
medulla oblongata *The inferior portion of the brainstem.*	kipande cha chini cha ncha ya ubongo
megacolon *Abnormal enlargement and dilatation of the colon.*	usiokuwa wa kawaida utvidgningen ya matumbo kubwa
meibomian cyst *An enclosed fluid collection along a sebaceous gland of the eyelid.*	ndogo uvimbe kwenye ukope
melancholia *Profound sadness.*	makubwa huzuni
melanoma *Malignant cancer, typically found in the skin.*	kufisha saratani ya ngozi
melena *The passage of black, tarry stools indicative of upper gastrointestinal bleeding.*	umwagaji damu kinyesi
melitis *Inflammation of the cheek.*	kiwasho cha shavu
member *Referring to an extremity (arm or leg).*	mkono au mguu
memory *Ability to remember.*	kumbukumbu
menarche *The time of the initial menstrual period.*	kwanza ya hedhi kipindi
meningeal *Referring to the dura mater, arachnoid and the pia mater.*	ngozi tatu zinazofunika ubongo na uti wa mgongo
meningitis *Inflammation of the meninges exhibited by fever, photophobia, nuchal rigidity and in severe cases coma and convulsions.*	ugonjwa sifa kwa shingo ugumu, homa, na wakati mwingine kukosa fahamu

English	Swahili
meniscus *A thin cartilage between joint surfaces.*	mfupa laini kwenye kiungo cha goti ambao una sura ya nusu mwezi
menopause *The time when menstruation ceases.*	wanakuwa wamemaliza kuzaa
menorrhagia *Abnormally large amount of menstrual blood.*	hali isiyo ya kawaida kubwa kiasi cha damu ya hedhi
menses *The blood and other material expelled from the uterus during menstruation.*	damu ya mwezi
menstrual cramps	zingizi
menstruation *Synonym of menses.*	mwezi; hedhi
mental *Cognitive or psychological.*	akili
mention, to *Refer to or allude to.*	kutaja
metacarpophalangeal *Referring to the metacarpus and the phalanges.*	pahali kidole cha mkono kinashikana na mkono
metrorrhagia *Uterine bleeding in normal amounts but at irregular intervals.*	kawaida kiasi cha hedhi lakini katika vipindi kawaida
microcephalic *A congenital deformity exhibited by an abnormally small head.*	hali isiyo ya kawaida kichwa ndogo
micrognathia *Abnormally small maxilla or mandible.*	hali isiyo ya kawaida ndogo taya
microscope *A instrument used to magnify and view small objects.*	darubini; hadubini
micturition *Synonym of urination.*	kukojoa
midwife *A person trained to assist in childbirth.*	mkunga
migraine *An episodic, unilateral headache accompanied by nausea.*	maumivu cha kichwa upande mmoja; kipandauso
mild *Slight, nominal.*	kali
milestone *An event indicative of a certain stage of development.*	hatua
minute *Something very small.*	dakika
mirror *A device used for reflecting an image.*	kioo
miscarriage *Spontaneous abortion.*	kuharibika kwa mimba
mite fever *Synonym of typhus fever.*	kimchango homa
mitochondria *Organelle found in cells responsible for energy production.*	pahali ndani ya chembechembe ambapo chckula huchomwa na kubadirishwa kuwa nguvu
moist *Damp or humid.*	unyevu
molar tooth *Any of the most posterior teeth bilaterally which includes 8 deciduous and usually 12 permanent teeth.*	gego
monitor *A person that observes a process or a monitoring device.*	mtazamaji
monocyte *A leukocyte with an oval nucleus and grey cytoplasm.*	monosaiti
monodiplopia *Double vision in only one eye.*	mara mbili maono katika jicho mmoja tu
mononucleosis *An infectious disease exhibited by malaise and lymphadenopathy.*	magonjwa ya kuambukiza na sifa ya unyonge na utvidgningen ya limfu nodi
monoplegia *Paralysis of a single limb.*	ulemavu wa mkono mmoja au mguu
morbidity *The state of disease.*	maradhi

93

English	Swahili
morgue *A room where deceased patients are housed until sent to a funeral home.*	mochari
moribund *Near death.*	karibu kifu
morning sickness *Nausea associated with pregnancy.*	ugonjwa wa asubuhi (kichefuchefu yanayohusiana na mimba)
mosquito net *A fine mesh fabric hung over a bed as a mosquito repellent.*	chandalua
motion sickness *Nausea associated with travel.*	ugonjwa mwendo
motor *Referring to muscles.*	kusogea
mourning *A period of grieving.*	maombolezo
mouth *The orifice on the lower part of the face.*	kinywa
mouthful *A large quantity of something in one's mouth.*	funda
mucus *A substance secreted by mucous membranes.*	belghamu
multigravida *A woman who has been pregnant more than once.*	mimba zaidi ya mara moja
multipara *A woman with more than one live births.*	zaidi ya mmoja kuishi kuzaliwa
mumble, to *To speak quietly and indistinctly.*	sema tirivyogo
mumps *A contagious viral disease that is exhibited by parotid swelling and puts males at risk for sterility. Also called epidemic parotitis.*	perema; matubwitubwi; machapwi
muscle *A band if fibrous tissue that can contract.*	misuli
muscle weakness *Decreased muscular function.*	udhaifu wa misuli
muscle, abdominal	misuli ya fumbatio
muscle, biceps	shavu la mkono
muscle, calf	shavu la mguu
muscle, deltoid	misuli ya bega
muscle, gluteus maximus	misuli ya matako
muscle, intercostal	misuli kati ya mbavu
muscle, latissimus dorsi	misuli ya mgongo wa juu
muscle, oblique	misuli mishazari
muscle, pectoral	misuli ya kifua
muscle, quadriceps	misuli wa paja
muscle, trapezius	misuli wa ukosi
mute *Refraining from or being speechless.*	bubu
myalgia *Muscle pain.*	maumivu ya misuli
mycosis *A disease caused by a fungal infection.*	ugonjwa unaosababishwa na fangasi
myelitis *Inflammation of the spinal cord.*	kiwasho cha uti wa mgongo

English	Swahili
myocardial infarction *The death of myocardial tissue as a result of an interruption in flow to the region supplied by a coronary vessel.*	mshtuko wa moyo
myocardium *The middle layer of the heart wall.*	misuli nyama ya moyo
myopia *Nearsightedness.*	nzuri karibu maono
myositis *Inflammation of muscle tissue.*	kiwasho ya misuli
nail *The hard surface on the dorsal surface of the toes or fingers.*	ukucha
name *A word by which a person is known.*	jina
nap *A brief sleep or catnap.*	usingizi mfupi
nappy *Diaper*	kiwinda
narcissism *Abnormally excessive self-interest.*	kujipenda
nasal mucus *Secretions coming from the nose.*	kamasi
nasogastric tube *A tube that is inserted into the nose with the distal tip in the stomach; it is used for irrigation or drainage of gastric contents.*	mrija wa kusafisha tumbo kuingizwa kupitia pua
nasopharyngeal *Referring to the nose and pharynx.*	akimaanisha pua na koo
nasopharynx *The part of the pharynx which lies superior to the soft palate.*	sehemu ya kishimo kilicho nyuma ya pua, kinywa na kikoromeo juu ya kaakaa laini
nausea *A feeling that one wants to vomit.*	kichefuchefu
navel *Umbilicus.*	kitovu
near *In close proximity.*	karibu
nebulizer *A device used for transforming a liquid into a fine mist for inhalation as in nebulized albuterol for an acute exacerbation of asthma.*	kifaa kwamba mabadiliko ya dawa kioevu katika ukungu kwa kuvuta pumzi
neck *The part of the body that connects the body to the head.*	shingo
neck, back of (nape) *Posterior aspect of the neck.*	kisogo; ukosi
necropsy *Synonym of autopsy.*	uchunguzi baada ya kifo
necrosis *The death of most of the cells of the affected part.*	hakuna mtiririko wa damu na sehemu ya kuoza mwili na ya baadae ya sehemu ambayo
need *A want or obligation.*	haja
needle biopsy *Use of a needle to aspirate body contents for microscopic or pathologic examination.*	tishu sampuli kwa kutumia sindano
needle holder *A surgical instrument used to grasp a needle during suturing.*	kifaa kutumika kushikilia sindano
needle *The slender cylindrical device attached to a syringe.*	sindano
negative *Contrary or opposing.*	hataki
nematode *An endoparasite belonging to the class of the Nemathelminthes including roundworms and threadworms.*	nematodi
neonate *The term for a newborn infant for the first four weeks.*	Watoto wachanga hadi nne umri wa wiki

English	Swahili
nephrectomy *Surgical removal of a kidney.*	Upasuaji kuondolewa figo
nephritis *A general term meaning inflammation of a kidney that is further categorized depending on the associated pathology.*	kiwasho ya figo
nephrolithiasis *A calculus in the kidney.*	kuwa na kujiwe figo
nephrolithotomy *Surgical removal of a renal calculus.*	upasuaji kuondolewa kwa jiwe figo
nephrotomy *Surgical incision of the kidney.*	chale upasuaji wa figo
nerve *A fibrous band made up of axons and dendrites that connects the nervous systems with other organs.*	mshipa wa fahamu
neurapraxia *Paralysis from nerve injury but no degeneration of the nerve.*	maumivu makali pamoja neva
neurectomy *Excision of a section of a nerve.*	upasuaji kuondolewa neva
neuritis *Inflammation of a nerve.*	kiwasho ya neva
neuropathy *Structural of pathologic changes of the peripheral nervous system.*	maumivu ya neva
neurosurgery *Surgery of the brain or spinal cord.*	upasuaji wa ubongo au uti wa mgongo
neutrophil *A polymorphonuclear leukocyte.*	nyutrofili
nevus *A benign, well-circumscribed growth of tissue of congenital origin.*	kuzalima alama
next *The following or upcoming.*	aidha
night blindness *Common term for nyctalopia, it refers to low vision with reduced illumination, often seen with Vitamin A deficiency.*	upofu wa usiku
night sweats *Profuse sweating at night occurring with tuberculosis among other conditions.*	kutokwa na jasho usiku
nightmare *An unpleasant or frightening dream.*	inatisha ndoto
nipple *The small projection on the breast thru which milk is secreted.*	chuchu; titi
nocturia *Urination at night.*	kukojoa usiku
nocturnal *Referring to events that happen at night.*	usiku
nodule *A small node in the skin of up to 1cm and in the lung up to 3cm.*	kifundo; kinundu
non-rebreather mask *A type of oxygen mask used to deliver a higher oxygen concentration.*	kifuniko cha uso kinachozuia hewa kutoka
nonpitting edema *Subcutaneous swelling that cannot be indented with compression.*	uvimbe kuwa haina kuondoka anatengeneza
noon *The 12 o'clock mid-day hour.*	mchana
nose *The midface protuberance used for smelling and breathing.*	pua
nose, blow the	penga kamasi
nosebleed *Common term for epistaxis.*	muhina
nostril *One of two openings in the nose used for air passage.*	tunda la pua
nulligravida *A woman who has never been pregnant.*	kamwe kuwa mjamzito
nullipara *A woman who has never given birth.*	kamwe kupewa kuzaliwa
numbness *Decreased sensation to tactile stimuli.*	ganzi
nurse *A person trained to care for the sick.*	mwaguzi; nesi
nursing care *The assessment and treatment provided by nurses.*	uguza
nutrition *The process of supplying food needed for growth.*	chakula bora

English	Swahili
nystagmus *Rapid involuntary movement of the eyes; it can be horizontal, vertical or rotary.*	haraka mwendo usio wa hiari ya macho
obesity *Having a body mass index over 30kilograms/meters squared.*	unene
obsolete *No longer in use; antiquated.*	kizamani
obstructed *To be blocked or halted.*	kuwa imefungwa
obtuse *Rather insensitive or hard to understand.*	butu
occiput *Back of the head.*	kogo
occlusion *A pathway that is blocked or obstructed.*	uzuiaji
ocular paralysis. *Paralysis of intraocular and extraocular muscles.*	kutokuwa na uwezo wa hoja macho
odiferous *Having an unpleasant or distinctive smell.*	ovundo
odontalgia *Tooth pain.*	maumivu ya meno
odontoid *A prominence on the second cervical vertebra on which the first cervical vertebra pivots.*	sehemu nyembamba inayojitokeza kwenye kifupa cha pili cha uti wa mgongo ambapo kifupa cha kwanza cha uti wa mgongo huzungukia
odor *A smell that is given off someone or something.*	harufu
odynophagia *Pain associated with swallowing.*	maumivu ya kuhusishwa na kumeza
offspring *One's children. (child)*	watoto (mtoto); mwana
ointment *A petroleum jelly based topical medication.*	dawa makao marashi
old age *A relative term for the period of advanced years.*	ukongwe
older *Being around more than compared with another.*	wakubwa
olecranon *The bony protrusion at the proximal ulna at the elbow.*	sehemu nyembamba upande wa juu kwenye mfupa mkubwa wa mkono kati ya kiko na kiwiko
olfactory *Referring to the sense of smell.*	akimaanisha hisia za harufu
oligodactyly *Presence of fewer than 5 digits on a hand or foot.*	wachache zaidi ya tano vidole juu mkono
oligohydramnios *Inadequate amount of amniotic fluid.*	kiasi kidogo ya maji yanayozunguka kijusi
oligomenorrhea *Infrequent menstruation or low volume menstrual flow.*	hali isiyo ya kawaida kiasi kidogo cha damu ya hedhi
oligotrophia or hypotrichosis *Less than normal amount of head/body hair.*	hali isiyo ya kawaida ndogo kiasi cha nywele mwili
oliguria *Abnormally low urine output.*	hali isiyo ya kawaida ndogo kiasi cha pato mkojo
omphalitis *Inflammation of the umbilicus.*	kiwasho ya kitovu
on going *Continuing,*	inayoendelea
oncologist *A physician specializing in the treatment of cancer.*	daktari wa kansa
onset *The beginning of an event.*	mwanzo
onychia *Inflammation of the toenail or fingernail matrix.*	kiwasho ya ukucha wa kidole cha mkono
onychomycosis *Fungal disease of the toenails or fingernails.*	vimelea wa magonjwa ya ukucha wa kidole cha mkono
onychophagia *Habitually chewing on one's fingernails.*	kutafuna ya ukucha wa kidole cha mkono

97

English	Swahili
oophorectomy *Surgical removal of an ovary.*	upasuaji kuondolewa kwa ovari
oophoritis *Inflammation of an ovary.*	kiwasho ya ovari
ooze, to *To slowly leak.*	kutona; kuvuja
operation *A surgical procedure.*	upasuaji
ophthalmia *Profound inflammation of the eye or its structures.*	kiwasho ya macho
ophthalmologist *A physician specializing in diseases of the eye.*	daktari wa macho
opium *An addictive drug derived from opium poppy; synthetic versions are used as analgesics.*	kasumba
optometrist *A person who practices optometry.*	daktari wa macho
oral *Relating to the mouth.*	mdomo
oral contraceptive *Tablet taken by mouth to prevent pregnancy.*	mdomo uzazi wa mpango
orally *By mouth. (verbally)*	kwa kinywa (kwa kunena)
orbit *The bony structure enclosing the eyeball.*	mfupa yanayozunguka jicho
orchialgia *Testicular pain.*	maumivu ya koko
orchidectomy *Synonym of orchiectomy; removal of one or both testes.*	upasuaji kuondolewa cha koko
orchitis *Inflammation of one or both testes.*	kiwasho ya koko
oropharynx *The portion of the pharynx between the soft palate and the superior aspect of the epiglottis.*	sehemu ya kichimo kilicho nyuma ya pua, kinywa na kikoromeyo kati ya kaakaa laini na ulimi mdogo
orthopedics *A surgical specialty concerned with treatment of skeletal problems.*	upasuaji maalum ya mifupa
orthopnea *The inability to breath comfortably except in the upright position.*	kupumua kwa shida wakati kuwekewa chali
orthostatic *Referring to the standing position. Orthostatic hypotension is low blood pressure in the standing position.*	chini ya shinikizo la damu katika nafasi ya kusimama
osteomyelitis *Inflammation of the bone or bone marrow because of a microorganism.*	maambukizi na kiwasho ya mfupa
osteoporosis *Loss of bone substance because the osteoblasts fail to produce bone matrix.*	hali ya kupoteza uguma wa mifupa
osteotomy *Creation of a surgical opening in bone.*	uundwaji wa ufunguzi upasuaji katika mfupa
otalgia *Ear pain.*	maumivu ya sikio
otitis externa *Inflammation of the middle ear*	kufura kwa sikio la ndani
otitis *Inflammation of the ear. (otitis media or otitis externa)*	kiwasho ya sikio
otomycosis *Fungal infection of the ear.*	maambukizi ya vimelea ya sikio
outdated *Something that has passed the expiration date.*	zilizopitwa na wakati
ovary *One of a paired of female reproductive glands containing oocytes.*	kifuko pahali ambapo mayai hutengenezewa ndani ya tumbo la mwanamke
overdose *An above normal dose of a medication.*	kuchukua zaidi ya kiasi kinachotakiwa cha dawa
overt *Not hidden.*	waziwazi
oviduct *The channel which an ovum passes from the ovary.*	mrija kuunganisha ovari ya mji wa mimba

ovulation *The release of an ova from the ovary.* — yai kuachiliwa kutoka kwa kifuko cha mayai ndani ya tumbo la mwanamke

owing to *On account of.* — kwa sababu ya

oxygen *A colorless, odorless gas with atomic number 8.* — oksijeni

pace *Consistent and continuous movement.* — kasi

pachydermia *An abnormally thick skin.* — hali isiyo ya kawaida nene ngozi

pain *Physical suffering or discomfort.* — maumivu

painless *Not painful.* — bila maumivu

palate *The roof of the mouth.* — kaakaa

palatoplegia *Paralysis of the palate.* — kupooza cha kaakaa

pallidectomy *Surgical resection of all or part of the palate.* — upasuaji kuondoa sehemu ya kaakaa

pallor *Unusually pale appearance.* — weupe

palm *The anterior aspect of the hand.* — kitanga cha mkono; kiganja

palpation *The assessment of the body with the use of one's hands.* — daktari kwa kutumia mikono yake bonyeza tumbo

palpebra, palpebrae *Eyelid, eyelids.* — kope, ukope

palpitation *Sensation of a forceful, rapid, irregular heartbeat present after exercise or with anxiety.* — kiherehere cha moyo

palsy *Paralysis that is usually associated with tremors.* — kupooza kuhusishwa na mitikisiko

pancreas *A gland that secretes digestive enzymes into the duodenum and insulin and glucagon into the blood.* — kongosho

pancreatectomy *Surgical excision of part or all of the pancreas.* — upasuaji kuondoa sehemu ya kongosho

pancreatitis *Inflammation of the pancreas.* — kiwasho ya kongosho

pandemic *When a disease is present over an entire region.* — gonjwa

panic attack *Sudden, profound anxiety.* — ishara ya hofu

papule *A small, well-circumscribed elevation of the skin.* — kijiwe

paracentesis *A procedure involving aspiration of fluid from the abdominal cavity.* — kuingiza sindano kupitia kwenye ngozi ya kuvuta maji kutoka ndani ya tumbo

paralysis *Inability to move one or more extremities.* — ugonjwa wa kupooza

paranasal *Situated adjacent to the nose.* — karibu na pua

paraplegia *Paralysis of the lower extremities.* — ulemavu wa miguu yote

pararectal *Adjacent to the rectum.* — karibu na mjiko

parasite *An organism that lives on or within another organism without benefit to the latter.* — kimelea

paresis *Incomplete paralysis.* — si kamili kupooza

paresthesia *An abnormal sensation usually described as pins and needles.* — ganzi

Parkinson's disease *A progressive neuromuscular disease exhibited by masklike facial expression, resting tremor, cogwheel rigidity and abnormal gait.* — magonjwa Parkinson

paronychia *Inflammation of the tissue bordering a fingernail* — kiwasho wa kidole karibu na ukucha

parturition *The process of giving birth.* — kujifungua

99

English	Swahili
passive *Not achieved through active effort.*	watazamaji tu
patella *The bone situated in the anterior portion of the knee.*	pia ya goti; kilegesambwa
patellectomy *Surgical excision of the patella.*	upasuaji kuondolewa cha kilegesambwa
pathogenesis *The course of a disease.*	mwenendo wa ugonjwa
patient *The client being treated for a medical or surgical condition.*	mgonjwa
pediatrician *Physician who is a specialist in pediatrics.*	daktari wa mtoto
pediculosis *Lice infestation.*	hali ya kuwa na chawa
pellagra *A deficiency in nicotinic acid exhibited by diarrhea and dermatitis.*	upungufu wa asidi nikotini ulioonyeshwa na kuhara na ugonjwa wa ngozi
pelvic inflammatory disease *Generally a bacterial infection affecting a woman with potential involvement of the uterus, fallopian tubes, ovaries and cervix.*	maambukizi ya kuwashirikisha ovari na mfuko wa uzazi
pemphigus *A skin disorder with large bullous lesions.*	hali ya ngozi na sifa ya malengelenge kubwa
penis *Male genital organ used for the transfer of sperm and elimination of urine.*	uume; mboo
perforation *Presence of a hole.*	kipenyo
pericardial tamponade *Decrease in systemic perfusion related to a collection of fluid in the pericardial space.*	hali ambapo sehemu iliyo kati ya moyo na ngozi inzungukao moyo hujazwa na maji ya mwili
pericarditis *Inflammation of the pericardium.*	kiwasho ya ngozi jirani moyo
pericardium *The structure enclosing the heart which contains a fibrous outer layer and serous inner layer.*	ngozi jirani moyo
perineal *Referring to the perineum.*	sehemu kati ya kuma na mkundu
perinephric *Around the kidney.*	jirani figo
perineum *The area between the anus and scrotum or anus and vulva.*	msamba
peripheral *Referring to an outward part or surface.*	pembeni
peritoneum *The serous membrane covering the abdominal organs and lining the abdominal walls. (utambi also means wick in Swahili)*	utambi
peritonitis *Inflammation of the peritoneum.*	kiwasho ya utambi
peritonsillar abscess	halula
personality *Qualities that form a person's unique character.*	utu
perspiration from armpit (or bad body odor)	adhifari
perspiration *The process of sweating.*	kutoka jasho
pertussis *Synonym for whooping cough.*	kifaduro
pes cavus *Excessive height of the longitudinal arch of the foot.*	hali isiyo ya kawaida ya juu mvungo wa wayo
pes planus *Medical term for flat foot.*	gorofa mvungo wa wayo
Peyronie's disease *Curvature of the penis during an erection due to plaque.*	uviringo ya uume wakati simika
phalanges *The long bones of the fingers or toes.*	mifupa ya vidole vya mikono ama vya miguu

English	Swahili
phantom limb pain *Pain sensed in an area where one has had an amputation as though the limb is still present.*	maumivu katika mguu kwamba imekuwa ulikatwa
pharmacist *A professional who prepares and sells medicine through various systems, including governmental organizations like the Veterans Administration.*	mchanganyaji dawa
pharmacy *A business that sells prescription medication.*	duka la madawa
pharyngitis *Inflammation of the pharynx.*	kiwasho ya koo
pharynx *The membranous cavity from the mouth to esophagus. (umio is sometimes used to describe esophagus at also the larynx)*	koo; umio
phobia *An profound fear of something.*	hofu kubwa ya kitu
photophobia *Abnormal sensitivity to light.*	usiokuwa wa kawaida usikivu kwa mwanga
physical exam *Examination of a client to assess their medical status.*	uchunguzi wa afya
physical therapy *Treatment of disease by heat, massage and exercise as opposed to medications.*	tiba ya mwili
physician *Medical practitioner.*	daktari; mganga
pia mater *The first layer of three covering the brain and spinal cord.*	sehemu ya ndani ya ngozi ifunikayo ubongo na uti wa mgongo
pill *A medicated tablet or capsule.*	tembe; dawa; vidonge
pillow *An encased fabric covering soft material used for a cushion.*	mito
pink eye *Common term for acute contagious conjunctivitis.*	kiwasho ya ngozi nyembamba inayofunika sehemu ya nje ya jicho ndani ya kope
pinworm *Common term for Enterobius vermincularis; a nematode worm that is a parasite.*	nematodi mdudu kwamba ni vimelea
placenta *The vascular tissue that nourishes a fetus through an umbilical cord.*	kondo ya nyuma
placenta praevia *A condition in which the placenta covers the cervical os.*	kondo ya nyuma isiyo mahali pake
placental abruption *Premature detachment of a normally situated placenta.*	kutenganisha kondo la nyuma na ukuta wa chungu cha mtoto
plantar *Referring to the bottom of the foot.*	wayo
plantar wart *A viral epidermal growth on the bottom of the foot.*	chunjua ya wayo
plaster cast *Use of gypsum impregnated gauze to immobilize fractured extremities.*	plasta
plethora *An excess of something.*	wingi
pleura *The serous membrane lining each lung.*	ngozi kati ya kwa kifua na mapafu
pneumocystis jiroveci pneumonia. *A pulmonary infection associated with AIDS. Formerly called pneumocystis carinii pneumonia*	Pneumocystis nimonia
pneumonectomy *Surgical excision of all or part of a lung.*	upasuaji kuondolewa yote au sehemu ya uvimbe
pneumonia *Inflammation of the lung due to an infection caused by a virus or bacterium.*	kamata; mkamba

English	Swahili
pneumothorax *Abnormal presence of air between the lung and chest wall.*	usiokuwa wa kawaida mbele ya hewa kati ya mapafu na ukuta kifua
poison *A substance that causes illness or death.*	sumu
poliomyelitis *An infectious viral disease exhibited by constitutional symptoms that can lead to quadriplegia.*	kiharusi
polydactyly *Congenital anomaly exhibited by more than 5 digits on the hands and/or feet.*	tangu kuzaliwa, hali ya sifa kwa kuwa na vidole zaidi ya tano kwa upande mmoja
polydipsia *Profound thirst.*	kiu isiyoisha
polysialia *Abnormal increase in saliva.*	usiokuwa wa kawaida ongezeko katika mate
polyuria *Abnormal increase in volume of urine excreted.*	kukojoa sana
popliteal fossa *The hollow in the posterior aspect of the knee joint.*	upande wa nyuma ya goti
port-wine mark *Also called nevus flammeus, it is a vascular anomaly characterized by purplish skin discoloration.*	zambarau kubadilika rangi ya ngozi
positive *Indicating the presence of something.*	chanya
post-term birth *An infant born after the normal length of pregnancy.*	watoto wachanga waliozaliwa baada ya kipindi kirefu kuliko kawaida ujauzito
posterior *Further back in position; opposite of anterior.*	nyuma
postictal *The period of time after a seizure.*	kipindi cha muda baada ya mshtuko wa kifafa
postpartum psychosis *A episode of abnormal thought or hallucinations following delivery.*	wazimu baada ya kujifungua
postpone, to *To delay.*	kuahirisha
potency *Strength or power.*	nguvu au uwezo
powder *Fine dry particles.*	uvumbi
preauricular *Anterior to the ear.*	mbele ya sikio
pregnancy *The period of being pregnant.*	uja uzito; mimba; himila
pregnant woman	mjamzito
premature *Occurring earlier than expected.*	mapema
premenstrual *Occurring prior to the onset of menstruation.*	kabla ya kuanza kwa hedhi
premenstrual syndrome *A cluster of emotional, behavioral, and physical symptoms that occur in the premenstrual phase of the menstrual cycle and resolve with the onset of menstruation.*	ishara za kuonyesha kuwa wakati wa damu ya kila mwezi umekaribia
prenatal *Referring to the time prior to birth.*	akimaanisha wakati kabla ya kuzaliwa
presbyacusia *An age related, progressive hearing loss.*	umri-kuhusiana na kusikia hasara
presbyopia *Farsightedness associated with aging.*	wenye kuona mbali
prescription *The action of prescribing a medication or treatment.*	cheti cha daktari
presenting symptom *The initial subjective complaint that initiated a visit.*	dalili awali
pressure dressing *A dressing used for compression to reduce bleeding.*	bendeji inatumika kuzuia kutokwa na damu

pressure ulcer *Loss in skin integrity due to a portion of the body being in the same position for too long and possibly other factors.*
kidonda kuwa matokeo kutoka kuwekewa kitandani kwa muda wa siku nyingi

prevent, to *To stave off or hinder.*
kukinga; kuzuia

priapism *A painful and abnormally prolonged erection.*
chungu ya muda mrefu simika

prickly heat *A rash with small vesicles that is pruritic and associated with a warm moist environment. Also called miliaria rubra.*
harara

primipara *A woman giving birth for the first time.*
mwananamke aliyezaa mara moja

problem *Difficulty or complaint.*
ugumu au malalamiko

proctectomy *Surgical excision of the rectum.*
upasuaji kuondolewa kwa njia ya haja kubwa

proctitis *Inflammation of the rectum.*
kiwasho ya njia ya haja kubwa

proglottis *Any segment of a tapeworm.*
sehemu yoyote ya tegu

prognosis *The likely course of a disease.*
makisio ya maendeleo ya ugonjwa

progressive *Developing gradually.*
maendeleo

prolapse of the umbilical cord *Refers to the umbilical cord protruding from the cervix during active labor.*
wakati kanda ya kitovu inatoka kabla ya mtoto wakati wa kuzaliwa

prolapse of the uterus *Eversion of the uterus through the vagina.*
mbenuko ya mfuko wa uzazi kwa njia ya uke

prolonged rupture of the membranes *Rupture of the membranes more than 24 hours before delivery.*
vunja chupa kwa zaidi ya saa 24

promontory *A protruding eminence.*
sehemu inayotokeza

pronation *Turning posteriorly. When the hand is pronated, it is turned medially until the palm is facing posteriorly (when the body was initially in the anatomic position).*
kugeuka fudifudi

prone *Lying with the abdomen and face downward.*
fudifudi; uso chini

prophylaxis *That which is done to prevent disease.*
tiba ya kuzuia maradhi

proptosis oculi *Synonym of exophthalmos; bulging of the eye.*
mbenuko wa jicho

prostate *A gland found in men that surrounds the neck of the urethra and bladder.*
tezi kibofu

prostatectomy *Surgical excision of the prostate.*
upasuaji kuondolewa tezi kibofu

prostatitis *Inflammation of the prostate gland.*
kuvimba kwa tezi kwa wanaume

prosthesis *An artificial body part. (above the knee) [below the knee]*
bandia mwili sehemu

prostitute *A person who exchanges goods or services for sex.*
malaya

prostration *Profound exhaustion.*
kusujudu

protein *A class of nitrogenous organic compound.*
protini

proteinuria *The presence of protein in the urine.*
mbele ya protini katika mkojo

provoke, to *To evoke or elicit.*
kukasirisha

proximal *Situated closer to the center of the body (opposed to that which is farther away, as in distal).*
kupakana

pruritus *A general term for conditions exhibited by itching.*
mchochota

psychology *The study of the human mind and emotions.*
elimu ya mawazo

English	Swahili
psychosis *A profound mental disorder that can include delusions and hallucinations.*	makubwa ya ugonjwa wa akili
ptosis *Drooping of the upper eyelid usually due to paralysis of the third cranial nerve.*	udhaifu ya ukope
puberty *The time when adolescents become capable of sexual reproduction.*	ubalehe
pubic hair *Hair present in the perineal area.*	uvuzi
pubis *The anterior inferior part of the hip bone on each side that articulates at the pubic symphysis.*	mfupa wa kinena
puerperium *The six week period after childbirth.*	sita kipindi cha wiki baada ya kujifungua
puffiness *Having a soft, swollen area.*	eneo dogo la uvimbe
pull, to *To exert force on something.*	kuvuta
pulmonary edema *Characterized by abnormal fluid buildup in the lungs.*	maji mkusanyiko ndani ya mapafu
pulmonary embolism *A sudden blockage of a lung artery frequently emanating from a blood clot in one's leg.*	kukoma kwa mapafu
pulmonary *Referring to the lungs.*	akimaanisha mapafu
pulp *The tissue filling the root canals of a tooth.*	sehemu laini katikati ya jino yenye hisia na mishipa ya damu
pulpitis *Dental pulp inflammation.*	kuvimba kwa sehemu nyororo, laini iliyoko katikati ya jino
pulse *The rhythmic throbbing of arteries felt at major vessels.*	kipigo cha mshipa wa damu
pupil *The opening at the center of the iris.*	kiini cha jicho
purpura *The presence of patches of ecchymosis or petechiae.*	zaidi ya mmoja kiraka ya akimosi
purulent *Referring to pus.*	akimaanisha usaha
pus *Thick yellow or green opaque liquid as seen with infection.*	usuha
pyorrhea *Emission of pus.*	chafu ya pus
pyrexia *Fever.*	homa
pyrosis *Synonym for heartburn.*	mchomo cha tumbo
pyuria *Presence of purulent material in the urine.*	usaha katika mkojo
quadriceps *The anterior thigh muscle composed of four muscles.*	misuli ya paja
quadriplegia *Paralysis of all four extremities.*	ulemavu wa mikono yote miwili na miguu yote
qualify *To become eligible by fulfilling a necessary standard.*	kuhitimu
quarantine *A place of isolation for infectious persons until it can be certain it is safe to let them mingle.*	karantini
querulousness *Whining or complaining.*	kunung'unika au kulalamika
quickening *Signs of life noted by a mother as the fetus moves.*	misogeo ya kwanza ya mtoto tumboni
quiescent *A time of inactivity.*	wakati wa shughuli hakuna
quiet *Making little or no noise.*	unyamavu
quinsy *Peritonsillar inflammation or abscess.*	jipu la kifuko au kiwasho
rabies *An infectious viral disease transmitted through the bite of a mammal. Symptoms include hydrophobia, pharyngeal spasms and hyperactivity.*	kalab

104

English	Swahili
radial *Referring to the radius.*	inayohusiana na mifupa mifupi na mipana ya mkono sehemu ya chini
radiation *1. The emission of energy in the form of electromagnetic waves. 2. Divergence from a common point.*	mnururisho
rage *Uncontrollable anger.*	ghadhabu
raise, to *To lift or bring up.*	kiunua
rape *Forced sexual relations.*	najisi
Rapid Eye Movement *The movement of a person's eyes during this period of sleep.*	haraka jicho harakati
rash *Exanthema or urticaria.*	uwati; upele
rat *A rodent that looks like a large mouse.*	panya
rat bite fever *As the name implies, it is a condition exhibited by fever, nausea and skin erythema after one is bitten by a rat.*	ugonjwa sifa kwa homa, kichefuchefu na upele
reaction *A response to an action.*	majibu
rebound *A term used to describe a type of tenderness found with peritonitis.*	duta
recollection *Memory.*	kumbukumbu
recover *(from a serious ailment)*	kupongea
rectal digital examination *Use of a gloved finger to assess the rectal vault.*	kuingizwa ya kidole ndani ya njia ya haja kubwa wakati wa mitihani ya matibabu
rectal *Referring to the rectum.*	akimaanisha ya njia ya haja kubwa
reduction *Return of a dislocated joint or fractured bone to its proper position.*	wakati mifupa inarudia uhusiano wa kawaida kila mfupa kitika sehemu yake
regardless of *Without consideration of.*	bila kujali
regurgitation *1. Backflow of blood in the heart. 2. Movement of gastric contents into the mouth.*	nyuma harakati ya damu katika moyo (1) cheu (2)
relapse *The return to a prior state of ill health.*	chamko
relapsing fever *A recurrent bacterial infection, with fever, caused by Spirochetes.*	matumizi ya kawaida ya maambukizi ya bakteria na homa
related to *Causally connected.*	kuhusiana na
relation *1. A person who has a blood or marriage connection.*	ukoo
reliable *Trustworthy.*	kuaminika
relief *Alleviation from pain or discomfort.*	unafuu
relieve, to (pain) *To make less severe.*	kufariji maumivu
REM (rapid eye movement) sleep *This period of sleep is associated with irregular respirations and heart rate, involuntary movements and dreaming.*	haraka jicho harakati wakati wa kulala
remission *A decrease in severity or a temporary resolution.*	kupungua kwa ukali
removal *The act of removing something.*	kuondoa
renal failure *Diminution of kidney function.*	kuharibika figo kazi
resection *The removal of tissue.*	kuondolewa kwa tishu
respirator *A device used to artificially ventilate a patient.*	kifaa kutumika kwa artificially kupumua kwa mgonjwa
respiratory arrest *Cessation of breathing.*	kukoma kupumua

105

English	Swahili
respiratory rate *The number of breaths per minute.*	kupumua kiwango cha
rest *Relaxation or respite.*	mapumziko
restless, to be *Wriggle or squirm. Extreme restlessness, tossing around in bed.*	gaagaa
retching *Spasm of the stomach without presence of gastric material.*	kokomoka
retractor *A device for pulling back tissue during surgery.*	chombo upasuaji kutumika kuvuta nyuma tishu
retrograde *Referring to backward movement.*	nyuma harakati
rheumatic pain *Pain related to rheumatoid arthritis.*	kang'ata
rheumatism *Any condition exhibited by inflammation and pain in the joints and muscles.*	baridi yabisi
rhinitis *A viral infection or allergic reaction exhibited by nasal mucosal inflammation.*	virusi maambukizi yanayoathiri pua kwa ndani
rhinoplasty *Plastic surgery performed on the nose.*	upasuaji akifanya kwenye pua
rhinorrhea *Abundant nasal mucosal drainage.*	belghamu kutoka pua
rhythm *The pattern or cadence.*	mahadhi
ribs *A series of curved paired boney articulations protecting the thorax. (In Swahili, ubavu is also used for "side", "hip" & rib.)*	mbavu
rickets *A condition exhibited by softening and bowing of the long bones; caused by Vitamin D deficiency.*	nyongea; chirwa
Rift valley fever *A human febrile illness that is an endemic disease in sheep, transmitted by mosquitos and direct contact and caused by a virus of the family Bunyaviridae.*	bonde la ufa homa
right *Correct, accurate (adjective)*	sahihi
right *Justice or fairness.(noun)*	haki
right *Opposite of left.*	kulia
right *Sure, agreed, OK (adverb)*	sawa
right-handed *Having a preference to use the right hand.*	kulia waliyopewa
rigor mortis *The normal stiffening of the muscles and joints that occurs a few hours after death.*	uthubutu wa mwili baada ya kifo
rinderpest *A viral disease primarily of cattle that is thought to have been eradicated as of 2001.*	sotoka
ringing in the ears *Common term for tinnitus.*	mvumo sikioni
ringworm *A fungal skin infection exhibited by pruritic well circumscribed patches on the scalp or feet.*	choa
risus sardonicus *A spasm of the facial muscles causing what appears to be a smile on one's face.*	jansi ya uso vinavyosababisha moja upande mmoja tabasamu
rodent *A gnawing mammal that includes rats and mice.*	panya
rosacea *Erythema of the cheeks and nose caused by chronic vascular and follicular dilation.*	rosasia
rotation *Movement around an axis.*	mzunguko
rotator cuff *The structure around the capsule of the shoulder joint formed by the infraspinatus, supraspinatus, teres minor and subscapularis muscles.*	kiungo wa bega
rubella *Also called German measles, it is characterized by a rash, fever, headache.*	rubela
rude *Ill-mannered.*	fidhuli

running suture *A method of sewing a wound in which there is a* punta
knot at each end and continuous otherwise.

rupia *A sign of tertiary syphilis in which there are bullae or*   ndogo malengelenge ambayo
vesicles formed on the skin that erupt and form crusts.   yanaonyesha kaswende

rupture *An instance of bursting suddenly.*   kuvunjika

ruptured membranes *Signal of onset of labor (in Swahili it is*   vunja chupa
commonly called "break the bottle")

sacrum *The bone formed by five fused vertebrae that is situated* kitokono; vifupa vitano vya
between the two hip bones.   mwisho vya uti wa mgongo
                                                                       vilvyoungamana

sadness *The state of being sad.*   sikitiko; masikitiko; sijiko

saline *A solution of sodium chloride.*   maji yenye chumvi

saliva *The watery liquid secreted by the salivary glands.*   mate

salivation *The process of secreting saliva.*   kinyaa ya mate

salpingitis *Inflammation of the fallopian tubes.*   kiwasho ya mrija kuunganisha
                                                                       ovari ya mji wa mimba

107

English-Swahili: salt-zymogen

English	Swahili
salt *Typically referring to sodium chloride.*	chumvi
sandfly fever *A febrile illness transmitted by a sandfly, from the genus Phlebotomus, and found in the Mediterranean.*	homa iletwayo na usubi
sanitary napkin *Cloth or synthetic material used to absorb menstrual blood.*	sodo; usafi kitambaa
saponify,to *The creation of soap from oil using an alkali.*	fanya kuwa sabuni
saturation *An amount, expressed in a percentage, that expresses the degree something is absorbed versus the maximal absorption possible.*	kueneza
saw *A hand or power-driven tool used for cutting.*	msumeno
scabies *A skin condition exhibited by intense pruritus and a macular rash commonly in the perineal and interdigital spaces.*	upele
scald *A burn injury from extremely hot water.*	unguza unaosababishwa na maji ya moto
scale *A device to check a person's weight.*	mizani
scalp *The skin covering the head except for the face.*	kichwani
scalpel *A knife used during surgery for incision of skin and tissue.*	koleo
scapula *Medical term for the shoulder blade.*	ncha (mwishoni) ya bega
scarlet fever *A condition caused by streptococci that is exhibited by fever and a bright red (scarlet) rash.*	homa ya vipele vyekundu
scatter *The degree to which repeated measurements differ.*	kutatawanya
scheme *A program or plan.*	mpango
schistosomiasis *A condition, sometimes known as bilharzia, which involves infestation with flukes of the genus Schistosoma.*	kichocho
schizophrenia *A chronic mental condition exhibited by delusions, hallucinations, and faulty perception.*	dhiki; ugonjwa sifa kwa wazimu, mtazamo udanganyifu, kuharibika
scissors *A cutting instrument with two blades, joined at the middle.*	mkasi
sclera *The white outer covering of the eyeball.*	sehemu nyeupe ya mboni
scleritis *Inflammation of the eyeball.*	kiwasho ya sehemu nyeupe ya mboni
sclerotomy *Surgical incision of the sclera.*	upasuaji chale ya sehemu nyeupe ya mboni
scolex *The front end of a tapeworm.*	sehemu ya mbele ya tegu
scoliosis *A lateral curvature of the spine.*	ikiwa na mgongo
scorpion	akrabu
scrape *An injury caused by having a body part rubbed against a rough surface.*	chubua; kwaruza
scratch *A long, narrow superficial wound.*	mkwaruzo
screening *An evaluation as part of a methodical study.*	uchunguzi

English	Swahili
scrofula *Cervical tuberculous lymphadenitis. (Mlezi also means guardian in Swahili)*	mti; mlezi
scrotum *The sac which contains the testes.*	mfuko wa pumbu; korodani
scurvy *A disease of vitamin C deficiency exhibited by bleeding gums.*	kiseyeye
secretion *The discharge of substances from cells or glands.*	kinyaa
sedative *A medication used to facilitate sleep or calm a person.*	dawa kutumika kwa ajili ya tulizo
see the doctor, to	kuona daktari
seizure *An episode of tonic/clonic movement noted in epilepsy.*	kifafa mshtuko
semen	madhii; shahawa
semen analysis *Evaluation of semen used as part of a fertility workup.*	uchambuzi wa shahawa
seminoma *A malignant tumor of the testis.*	saratani ya korodani
senility *The process of being senile.*	uzee
sensation *A perception when one is touched.*	kuhisi kugusa ya mwingine
sepsis *A condition exhibited by overwhelming inflammation due to infection.*	hali inayoletwa na kuongezeka kwa viini au sumu kwenye damu
septicemia *A systemic disease in which microorganisms or their toxins are in the blood stream.*	sumu kwenye damu
septum *A wall separating two chambers, the nasal septum for example.*	vya tenganisho;
sequela *A medical problem related to an initial injury or disease.(late sequelae)*	baadae ya matibabu tatizo kuhusiana na ugonjwa wa awali
sequestrum *Necrotic bone present in an injured or diseased bone.*	wafu mfupa katika mifupa awali kujeruhiwa
serial *In a series.*	katika mfululizo
serum *The fluid that isolates out when blood coagulates.*	sehemu yenye maji katika damu
severe *Intense or very great.*	kali
sex *Gender.*	jinsia
sexual intercourse *The act of copulation.*	kulalana
sexually transmitted disease (STD) *A condition one obtains from another during sexual relations.*	ugonjwa unaoambukiza kwa njia ya kulalana
shake, to *To tremble uncontrollably.*	kuwa kitapo
sharp (pain) *When describing pain, a piercing sensation.*	mkali
sheath *A covering.*	ala
sheet (bed) *A rectangular fabric covering a bed.*	shuka ya kitanda
shellfish *An aquatic shelled crustacean or mollusk.*	kombe
shin *Refers to the anterior tibial region.*	muundi
shingles *A reactivation of herpes zoster.*	mkanda wa jeshi
shiver *A trembling.*	kitapo
shock *A condition characterized by systemic hypoperfusion.*	chini sana shinikizo la damu
shock *Surprise or astonishment. (startled)*	bumbauzi; (mshtuko)
shoe *Article of clothing worn on each foot.*	kiatu
shortening *Notable for having a shorter length.*	kufupisha
shoulder *The joint were the scapula joins the clavicle and humerus. (right shoulder, left shoulder)*	bega

109

English	Swahili
shunt *An alternate path for blood or fluid.*	njia tofauti na kusafiri kwa ajili ya damu au maji ya
sibling *A brother or sister. (younger sibling)*	ndugu (mdogo)
sickness *Illness or a state of disease.*	ugonjwa
side *A position medial or lateral to center.*	upande
side effect *An expected but unwanted effect of a medication.*	inayojulikana lakini isiyopaswa madhara ya dawa
sigh *A long deep exhalation that expresses an emotion, as in relief.*	wanaougua
silent *Absence of noise or no indication of something.*	nyamavu
simultaneous *Occurring at the same time.*	samtidiga
single *Not married.*	si ndoa
single *Only one.*	moja tu ya
sinusitis *Inflammation of the sinuses.*	kiwasho ya pango katika sehemu yo yote mwilini
sip, to *To slowly take small drinks of a fluid.*	kunywa kiasi kidogo polepole
site *Location.*	mahali
size *The dimensions of something.*	ukubwa
skeletal traction *Use of a pulley system to reduce a fracture.*	kuvuta ya mfupa kutibu mfupa uliovunjika (kutumia mfumo wa kapi)
skeleton *Internal bony framework.*	kiunzi cha mifupa
skin *Flesh.*	ngozi
skin disease that causes red spots	kipwepwe
skin fold *An overlapping of skin formed by subcutaneous tissue.*	mkunjo ya ngozi
skin rash *Dermal exanthema.*	vipele ngozini
sleep *A nap or a snooze. (deep sleep)*	usingizi (usingizi mzito)
sleep apnea *Episodic apnea during sleep that is exhibited by daytime symptoms of fatigue, difficulty concentrating and sleepiness.*	ugonjwa sifa kwa vipindi ya kukoma kinga wakati wa kulala
sleeping sickness *Also called Trypanosomiasis, this disease is caused by a parasitic protozoa and transmitted by the tsetse fly.*	malale
slight *Minor or small.*	kidogo
sling *A device used to give support to an injured extremity.*	kombeo
slow *Unhurried.*	polepole
sludge *A viscous fluid.*	kioevu nene sana
slurring *Indistinct yet comprehensible speech.*	kuzungumza ambayo nai vigumu kuelewa lakini kueleweka
smallpox *Variola.*	ndui
smegma *A thick curdled secretion found around the clitoris and the prepuce.*	kinyaa kupatikana katika kinembe na ngovi; pumba
smoke, to *To inhale on a cigarette.*	kuvuta (sigara)
snake (snake venom)	nyoka (sumu ya nyoka)
sneeze, to *To suddenly expel air from the nose and mouth because of nasal irritation. (a sneeze)*	piga chafya (chafya)
sniff,to *Short, rapid nasal inhalation. (or to smell)*	kunusa

snore, to *To snore or grunt while breathing during sleep. (a snore)*	kukoroma (mkoromo)
snuff *Chewing tobacco.*	ugolo
soap *A compound made with fats/oils and an alkali; it is used for washing.*	sabuni
sob, to *To cry uncontrollably.*	kulia
socket *An anatomical hollow that is part of an articulation. (eyeball socket)*	tundu (tundu la jicho)
socks *Worn on the feet before one puts on shoes.*	soksi
sodium chloride *A colorless, crystalline compound; also table salt.*	chumvi
soft *Easy to mold or compress.*	laini
sole of foot *Common term for plantar aspect of the foot.*	wayo
somnambulism *Sleepwalking.*	usingizi-kutembea
somnolence *Drowsiness.*	kusinzia
sorcery *Black magic or voodoo.*	ulozi; uchawi
sore throat *Common term for pharyngitis.*	maumivu ya koo
sound *Vibrations that travel through air and are heard when reaching the ears.*	sikitiko; msiba; buka
sour *An acid or bitter taste.*	chachu
span *A distance between two objects.*	umbali kati ya vitu
spasm *An involuntary contraction of muscles.*	kiharusi
specific *Clearly defined.*	maalum
specimen *A sample for medical testing.*	damu au mkojo sampuli
speculum *A device used to open a canal for inspection. (vaginal speculum)*	matibabu chombo kutumika kukagua uke
speech *Oral articulation.*	nena
speech therapist *A person trained to assist people with speech and language disorders.*	mtaalamu katika matatizo ya lugha na akizungumza
sperm *Short term for spermatozoon.*	manii
spermatogenesis *The production of spermatozoa.*	uzalishaji wa manii
spermicide *A substance capable of killing sperm.*	kemikali cha uwezo wa kuua manii
sphygmomanometer *Device for measuring blood pressure.*	kipimadamu
spinal cord abscess *A localized collection of purulent material in or adjacent to the spinal cord.*	jipu ya uti wa mgongo
spinal cord *The bundle of nerves that with the brain comprise the central nervous system.*	uti wa mgongo
spine *The spinal column or a thorny protrusion.*	mgongo
spit *A term used to describe saliva that is ejected from the mouth.*	mate
spleen *The visceral organ that is involved with production and removal of blood cells.*	wengu; bandama
splenectomy *Surgical excision of the spleen.*	upasuaji kuondoa wengu
splenomegaly *An abnormally enlarged spleen.*	usiokuwa wa kawaida utvidgningen ya wengu
splint *A rigid support used to immobilize and extremity.*	gango

111

English	Swahili
splinter *A small, thin object; usually refers to the object being imbedded in the body.*	kibanzi
sponge *Sterile fabric used to soak up fluid during surgery.*	sifongo kutumika katika upasuaji
spontaneous *Occurring without provocation.*	zinazotokea bila ya uchochezi
sprain *A joint injury without fracture.*	kuraruka au kukazika kwa misuli au nyama
sputum *A mixture of respiratory tract secretions and saliva.*	kohozi; belghamu
squeeze, to *To apply pressure.*	minya
squint, to *To look at something with the eyes partially closed.*	kengeza
stab wound *An injury occurring with a sharp object.*	dunga jeraha
stabbing pain *A sharp piercing quality to pain.*	kichomi
stagger, to *To walk in an unsteady fashion.*	yumba
stamina *Ability to maintain physical or mental exertion for a long period.*	imara
stammer,to *The impulse to repeat the first letter of words and involuntary pauses while speaking.*	kigugumizi
stand *To stop or to be upright*	simama
standing *Position or status.*	msimamo au hali
starvation *Death related to starvation.*	njaa
stasis *Lack of movement.*	ukosefu wa harakati
steatorrhea *Excrement with an abnormally high fat content.*	kuhara mafuta
stenosis *Narrowing of an orifice.*	nyembamba ya kitundu
stereognosis *The ability to identify an object by touch.*	uwezo wa kutambua kitu kwa kugusa
sterile *1. Infertile 2. Refers to equipment that is free of contamination.*	si rutuba (1), kuzaa
sternum *Commonly called the breast bone, it consists of the corpus, manubrium and xiphoid process.*	mfupa wa kidari
stiff *Not easily bent.*	si rahisi kwa mara
stillborn *Refers to a newborn that died in utero.*	mtoto anayezaliwa akiwa mfu
sting *A small puncture as in a bee sting.*	uma
stomach *Organ of digestion between the esophagus and small bowel.*	tumbo
stomach cramps *Sensation of muscle contraction in the epigastric area.*	kichomi ya tumbo
stomach ulcer *Gastric ulcer.*	vidonda tumbo; alasi
stool *Feces, excrement.*	kinyesi
stool, watery with mucous	malendalenda
strain *As in a muscle strain.*	mshtuko
strength *Force, might or vigor.*	nguvu; uwezo
stress *Strain or pressure.*	mkazo
stretcher *A device used to carry a patient in the supine position.*	machela
stricture *A narrowing of a canal or duct.*	nyembamba ya mfereji
stridor *An abnormal, high-pitched, musical sound caused by an obstruction in the larynx or stenosis of the vocal cords.*	sauti za juu zinazotokana na kufinyika kwa njia za hewa
stroke *Common term for cerebrovascular accident.*	kiharusi

112

English	Swahili
strong *Having the power to move heavy objects.*	nguvu
stump *Term used to designate what remains of an amputated extremity.*	gutu la mguu au mkono
stupor *A reduced level of consciousness.*	uzito wa akili
stuttering *Involuntary repetition of the first consonant.*	babaika
sty *Also called hordeolum externum, it is inflammation of the sebaceous gland of an eyelash.*	chokea
subacute *A stage between acute and chronic.*	kali kiasi
subarachnoid *The layer of the brain covering between the arachnoid and pia mater.*	ile ngozi ya katikati kabisa kati ya zile tatu zizungukazo ubongo na uti wa mgongo
subdural *The area between the dura mater and the arachnoid membrane.*	chini ya ngozi nyembamba ifunikayo ubongo na uti wa mgongo
sublingual *Situated under the tongue.*	chini ya ulimi
submaxillary *Situated below the maxilla.*	chini ya taya
subungual *Under a fingernail or toenail.*	chini ya kucha za mikono au miguu
suck, to *As in, to suction fluid.*	fyonza
suckle, to *An infant taking to his mother's nipple.*	nyonyesha
suffer, to *To be affected by an illness or sickness.*	kuteseka
suffocation *To die from a lack of air or inability to breathe.*	kukosekana hewa
sugar *A sweet crystalline substance made from a plant such as sugar cane.*	sukari
suicide *To kill oneself intentionally.*	kujiua makusudi
superior *In a position above something else.*	juu
supine *Flat on one's back.*	kingalingali
supplies *Stock or reserves.*	vifaa
suppository *A delivery system for medication placed in an orifice.*	dawa kutolewa katika mkundu au uke
suppuration *Formation of purulent material.*	tunga usaha
surgeon *A physician who performs surgery.*	daktari kwa upasuaji
surname *One's given "last" name that generally changes for women upon marriage to that of the man's surname.*	jina
sustain, to *To keep or maintain.*	kuendeleza
suture *Thread used for sewing together a wound.*	mshono wa kuziba jeraha
swab *An absorbent material used for cleaning wounds or applying ointment.*	shashi ya pamba
swallow, to *To cause something to pass down the esophagus.*	kumeza
sweat *Moisture exuded through the pores of the skin.*	jasho; hari
sweat, to *The action of releasing moisture through pores of the skin.*	tokwa na jasho
swelling *An abnormal enlarged from fluid collection.*	uvimbe
swollen (distended) abdomen	kuvimba tumbo
symmetry *Being equally bilaterally.*	ulinganifu
symptom *A physical feature that is characteristic of disease.*	dalili
syncope *Sudden loss of consciousness.*	ghafla kupoteza fahamu

English	Swahili
synovial fluid *The fluid that surrounds, for example, the knee within a capsule.*	ugiligili ya viungo (katika viungo kati ya mifupa)
syphilis *A infectious disease caused by Treponema pallidum that causes a painless penile ulcer in the primary stage but can lead to irreversible brain damage in the untreated tertiary stage.*	kaswende; sekeneko
syringe *A device used for administering medication through various routes.*	sindano; sirinji
syrup *A thick sweet liquid.*	asali
systolic *Referring to systole or that which occurs during systole.*	nguvu ipimwayo wakati moyo unapokuwa katika hali ya kusongana unapopiga
tablespoon *An eating utensil that holds 15milliliters of fluid.*	kijiko kikubwa
tablet *A small disk of a compressed solid substance.*	tembe; dawa; vidonge
tachycardia *Heart rate higher than physiologic normal.*	kiwango cha moyo zaidi ya 100 mapigo kwa dakika
tachypnea *Breathing faster than normal.*	kupumua kiwango cha juu ya kawaida
take medication, to	kunywa dawa
talipes equinovaro *Medical term for what is commonly known as club foot.*	kiguu
talus *The most superior tarsal bone that articulates with the tibia.*	mfupa wa kifundo cha mguu
tape measure *A long length of tape, marked at intervals for measuring.*	kifaa kwa kupima
tapeworm *A parasitic, intestinal flatworm.*	tegu
tarantula *A large hairy spider found mainly in the tropics.*	bui
target *An objective towards which efforts are directed.*	lengo
taste *Sensation of flavor perceived in one's mouth.*	ladha
tattoo *A design made by inserting indelible ink into the skin.*	tojo
tear *As in a vaginal tear after childbirth.*	pasuka
tears Fluid expelled from the eyes during crying.	machozi
teaspoon *A measure instrument that holds 5 milliliters of fluid.*	kijiko kidogo
temperature *The degree of internal heat in a person's body.*	ndani ya joto la mwili; halijoto
temple *The temporal fossa superior to the zygomatic arch.*	panja
tendinitis *Inflammation of a tendon.*	kufura kwa nyama nyembamba iunganishayo mifupa na misuli
tendon *Fibrous tissue that connects muscle to bone.*	ukano
tepid *Lukewarm.*	vuguvugu
terminal illness *A disease with no viable treatment with death being inevitable.*	ugonjwa kwamba itasababisha kifo
testicle *One of a pair of organs in the male scrotum that produces sperm.*	pumbu; kende
testicular torsion *Rotation of the spermatic cord resulting in testicular ischemia.*	makende yanapojipinda ndani ya ule mfuko wake
tetanus *A condition caused by Clostridium tetani which produces spasm and rigidity of voluntary muscles.*	pepopunda
thermometer *A device used to measure temperature.*	kipimajoto
thigh *The body region between the inguinal crease and knee.*	paja
thin *Lean or slender.*	embamba

English	Swahili
thirst *The desire to drink.*	kiu
thoracotomy *Surgical incision of the thorax.*	upasuaji chale ya kifua
thorax *The part of the body between the neck and abdomen.*	kifua
throat *The anterior aspect of the neck.*	koo
throb, to *The beat with strong regular rhythm.*	puma
thrush *Candida albicans*	kimenomeno
thumb *The first digit of each hand.*	kidole gumba
thyroid *A gland in the neck that secretes hormones regulating metabolism.*	tezi ya kikoromeo
thyroidectomy *Surgical resection of all or part of the thyroid.*	upasuaji kuondolewa tezi ya kikoromeo
tibia *The larger of two long bones in the lower leg.*	mfupa mkubwa katika sehemu ya chini ya mguu
tic *Periodic spasmodic facial muscle contractions.*	shtuko cha misuli usoni
tick bite	kumbwe cha papasi
tick-borne fever *A relapsing fever caused by a spirochete of the genus Borrelia.*	homa ya papasi
tickle, to *To lightly touch a person to cause one to laugh.*	tekenya
tidal volume *The amount of air inspired with each breath. One can set a ventilator to deliver a preset number of milliliters of oxygenated air with each breath.*	kiasi cha hewa ambacho mtu anapumua mara moja anapovuta pumzi katika hali ya kuwaida
tinea barbae *Ringworm on the face in the region a man shaves.*	choa ya uso
tinea capitis *Ringworm of the scalp, a fungal infection.*	bato
tinea corporis *Ringworm of the body, a fungal infection.*	choa ya mwili
tinea cruris *Ringworm in the inguinal region, a fungal infection.*	choa ya kinena
tinea *Medical term for ringworm.*	choa
tinea pedis *Ringworm of the feet, a fungal infection.*	nyungunyungu
tingling *Prickling or stinging sensation.*	sisimka
tinnitus *Medical term for ringing in the ears. It is associated with Meniere's syndrome among other conditions.*	mvumo sikioni
tired *Fatigued.*	uchovu
toe *Any of the digits of of the feet.*	kidole cha mguu
toenail *The nail at the tip/dorsal aspect of each toe.*	ukucha wa kidole cha mguu
tongs *A medical device used for holding or grasping.*	koleo
tongue *The fleshy muscular organ of the mouth.*	ulimi
tonsil *A rounded mass of lymphoid tissue, most commonly referring to the pharyngeal tonsil.*	tezi cha koo
tonsillitis *Inflammation of the tonsils.*	uvimbemchu ngu wa kifuko; kimio
tooth *One of a set of hard, bony enamel coated structure in the jaw.*	jino
toothache *Dental pain.*	kuumwa na jino
toothless *Edentulous.*	asiye na meno
toothless person	kibogoyo
torsion *Refers to twisting. Testicular torsion is the twisting of the spermatic cord that can lead to ischemia and gangrene of the testicle.*	uvimbemchu ngu wa kifuko
torso *The trunk of the body.*	kiwiliwili

115

English	Swahili
torticollis *A condition exhibited by the head being turned to one side continuously.*	hali ya sifa na kichwa kuwa akageuka katika mwelekeo mmoja kuendelea
touch *Tactile stimulation.*	gusa
tourniquet *A device tied tightly around an extremity to diminish blood flow or blood loss.*	kisongo
toxin *A poison of plant or animal origin.*	sumu; liga
trachea *The ringed canal between the pharynx and bronchi.*	umio wa pumzi
tracheitis *Inflammation of the trachea.*	kiwasho ya umio wa pumzi
tracheostomy *Creation of a surgical opening in the trachea so a tube could be placed in the trachea.*	upasuaji viumbe wa ufunguzi katika umio wa pumzi
trachoma *An infection of the cornea and conjunctiva caused by Chlamydia.*	maambukizi ya konea unasababishwa na Klamidia
tranquilizer *A medication used to diminish anxiety.*	dawa kutumika kwa kupunguza wasiwasi
transdermal *Through the skin.*	kupitia kwenye ngozi
transfusion *Administration of blood products intravenously.*	utawala wa damu ndani ya vena
transient ischemic attack *Cerebral ischemic changes resulting from transitory hypoperfusion.*	kupooza kwa muda mfupi
transplant,to *To move a body part from one location to another.*	atika
trauma *A physical injury or emotional shock.*	kiwewe
traumatic asphyxia *Cyanotic asphyxia due to trauma. Extravasation of blood into the skin and conjunctivae caused by a sudden increase in venous pressure from a crush injury.*	kufinywa kwa kfua kutokana na jeraha
treat, to *Medical care one receives for illness or injury.*	tibiwa
tremor *Involuntary contraction and relaxation of small muscle groups.*	tetemeko
trench mouth *Inflammation and ulceration of the gingivae.*	kiwasho na maambukizo of the ufizi
trendelenburg position *Position in bed in which the head is lower than the feet.*	hali ambapo kichwa cha mgonjwa huinuliwa juu ya moyo hasa kwa kusaidia kutibu kuzilai
trichinosis *A disease caused by meat infected by Trichinella spiralis causing fever and gastrointestinal effects.*	ugonjwa unaosababishwa na kula nyama ya kuambukizwa, ulioonyeshwa na homa na ugonjwa wa tumbo
triplets *Three infants born during one birth.*	watoto watatu waliozaliwa mimba moja
trismus *Commonly called lockjaw, it is a spasm of the muscles supplied by the trigeminal nerve and is an early symptom of tetanus.*	pepopunda
trivial *Of little importance or value.*	dogo
truss *A synthetic device for containing a hernia within the abdomen.*	kifaa kutumika kutoa msaada kwa ajili ya ngiri
trypanosomiasis *A disease caused by a protozoa of the genus Trypanosoma that can cause sleeping sickness and Chagas' disease.*	malale
tsetse fly *An insect that transmits the protozoa trypanosoma and can cause sleeping sickness.*	chafuo; pange

English	Swahili
tuberculosis *Any infectious disease caused by Mycobacterium.*	kifua kikuu
tuberosity *A protuberance. For instance the iliac tuberosity is a prominence on the surface of the ilium.*	mbenuko
tularemia *An infectious disease caused by Francisella tularensis. The symptoms range from mild constitutional complaints to septic shock.*	maumivu au ugonjwa unaoletwa na minni vinavyoenezwa na kupe
tumor *A benign or malignant overgrowth of tissue.*	tezi
twins *Two infants born at the same birthing.(identical twins)*	pacha (pacha fanani)
two times *One action being done on two occasions.*	mara mbili
tympanic membrane *The membrane between the external and middle ear.*	kiwambo cha sikio
tympanoplasty *Restoration of the tympanic membrane's continuity.*	upasuaji matengenezo ya kiwambo cha sikio
typhoid fever *A condition caused by ingestion of food or water containing salmonella typhi that is exhibited by fever and abdominal signs and symptoms.*	homa ya matumbo
typhus fever *A rickettsiae infection exhibited by rash, fever, headache and myalgia.*	Maambukizi Rickettsiae ulioonyeshwa na upele, homa na kuumwa na misuli, na maumivu ya kichwa
ulcer *A concave wound caused by a break in the integrity of skin or mucous membrane. (duodenal ulcer)*	donda
umbilical cord *The stalk between the placenta and the unborn infant.*	kitovu
umbilical tape *Material used to tie off the umbilical cord prior to cutting it after the baby is born.*	uzi wa kufungia kitovu
umbilicus *The scar that denotes the end of the umbilical cord.*	kitovu
unconsciousness *Unable to respond to sensory stimuli.*	bila fahamu
under; infra *Sometimes used when indicating a patient is "under treatment" for a condition (active treatment).*	chini ya
underlying *Causative, unexposed, or fundamental.*	misingi
undulant fever *Wave-like variations in the fever, going from very high to normal and back again, as seen in Brucellosis.*	homa kiwimbi
unexpected *Unforeseen.*	si inatarajiwa
unknown *Uncertain or undisclosed.*	haijulikani
upper limb *Referring to either arm.*	ama mkono
upright *Vertical or standing.*	wima
ureter *The conduit between each kidney and the urinary bladder.*	mrija kutoka figo na kibofu cha mkojo
ureterectomy *Surgical resection of one or both ureters.*	upasuaji kuondolewa kwa mrija kutoka figo na kibofu cha mkojo
ureteritis *Inflammation of the ureter.*	kiwasho ya mrija kutoka figo na kibofu cha mkojo
urethra *The canal connecting the urinary bladder with the outside of the body.*	mrija wa kutoa mkojo nje kutoka kibofu
urethritis *Inflammation of the urethra.*	kiwasho ya mrija wa kutoa mkojo nje kutoka kibofu
urethroplasty *Surgical repair of the urethra.*	upasuaji matengenezo ya mrija wa mkojo
urgency *Emergency or priority.*	uharaka

117

English	Swahili
urinal *Device used by men to void while in bed or sitting.*	chomba cha kukojolea
urinalysis *Chemical and microscopic examination of the urine.*	darubini ya uchunguzi wa mkojo
urinary bladder *The organ collecting urine from the ureters prior to discharge via the urethra.*	kibofu cha mkojo
urinary incontinence *Involuntary micturition.*	mkojo sababu ya udhaifu
urinary retention *Inadequately emptying the bladder.*	kutoweza kukojoa
urine *The fluid concentrated by the kidneys and expelled via the urethra.*	mkojo
urticaria *A diffuse pruritic macular rash, caused by an allergy.*	kueneza kinyevu na upele unasababishwa na mzio mmenyuko
usual *Typical or normal.*	kawaida
uterine bleeding *Bleeding that emanates from the uterus.*	damu kutoka mji wa mimba
uterus *The hollow organ in the female pelvis where a fertilized ovum embeds and grows.*	mji wa mimba
uvula *A fleshy pendent at the back of the soft palate.*	kidaka tonge; kimio
uvulectomy *Excision of the uvula.*	upasuaji kuondolewa kwa kidaka tonge
uvulitis *Inflammation of the uvula.*	kiwasho ya kidaka tonge
vaccination *The act of receiving a vaccine.*	chanjo ya kuzuia ungonjwa
vaccine *A solution of attenuated microorganisms given to prevent or treat a disease.*	chanjo
vaccine certificate *A document that denotes what vaccines have been received by the holder.*	chanjo cheti
vagina *The canal in a female that extends from the vulva to the cervix.*	uke
Valsalva's maneuver *A technique in which one attempts to exhale with the mouth and nose closed; this equalizes pressure in the ears.*	kulazimisha pumzi kwa njia ya kufunga mdomo, pua na kidakatonge ili kufanya moyo kupiga polepole
varicella *A virus that causes chickenpox and shingles. Also called herpes zoster.*	tetekuwanga
varicocele *A cluster of varicose veins in the scrotum.*	kufura kwa vena za pumbu
vascular *Referring to a blood vessel.*	enye mishipa ya damu
vasoconstriction *The process of making the blood vessels smaller which increases blood pressure.*	mshipa inakuwa miembamba
vasodilatation *The process of making the blood vessels larger which decreases blood pressure.*	mshipa inapanuka
vein *A vessel carrying blood back toward the heart.*	vena
venereal disease *A condition transmitted via sexual intercourse.*	ugonjwa wa zinaa
venereal wart *Common term for condyloma acuminatum.*	chunjua wa zinaa
venom (snake) *A term used to describe the toxin injected via a bite or sting.*	sumu ya nyoka
ventilation *The movement of air into the lungs; generally meant to suggest by an artificial process.*	pisha hewa safi
ventral *Referring to the underside but in humans, a ventral hernia, for example, refers to an abdominal hernia.*	mbele
ventricle *1. One of two chambers of the heart. 2. The four inter-connected cavities in the center of the brain.*	kifuko cha moyoni; upande wa chini wa kila nusu ya moyo

English	Swahili
ventricular fibrillation *Chaotic and ineffective ventricular contractions.*	kutetemeka kwa vifuko vyo moyo
ventriculography *Roentgenography of the ventricles after administration of contrast media.*	vena ndogo
verruca *A hyperplastic epidermal lesion, sometimes referred to as plantar wart.*	chunjua
vertebra *A term for each bone surrounding the spine.*	pingili ya mgongo
vertebral column *The cervical, thoracic and lumbar vertebrae.*	uti wa mgongo
vertex *The crown of the head.*	utosi
vertigo *A sensation of imbalance with many possible causes.*	kizunguzungu; gumbizi
vesicle *A blister.*	lengelenge
viable *Referring to a fetus that can survive childbirth.*	uwezo wa kuishi
viscous *Having a thick, sticky consistency.*	nene na nata uthabiti
vision *State of being able to see.*	maono
vision, blurred *Haziness of the visual field.*	kiwaa
vitiligo *The appearance of non-pigmented white patches on otherwise normal skin; hair is usually white in the affected areas.*	madoa meupe juu ngozi
vitreous *Glass appearance; used to describe the vitreous body of the eye.*	kitu kama majimaji kilichojaa kwenye macho
vocal cords *Paired folds of mucous membranes stretched across the larynx.*	mijadala kamba
voice *The sound produced through the larynx and out the mouth.*	sauti
voiding *The act of urinating.*	kukojoa
volunteer *A person who performs work without expecting compensation.*	kujitolea
volvulus *Twisting of the bowel leading to obstruction and sometimes perforation.*	kusokoteka kwa utumbo
vomit *The gastric contents that are expelled through the mouth.*	matapishi
vomit, to *To expel gastric contents out the mouth.*	kutapika
waddling gait *Walking in short steps in a swaying fashion.*	kutembea katika hali ile ile kama bata
walker *A metal frame used to facilitate walking.*	chuma kifaa kutumika kuwezesha kutembea
ward *A section of a hospital where patients reside.*	chumba katika hospitali
wart *A flesh colored growth that is also called verruca.*	chunjua
wart on clitoris	kinyakazi
wasp *Any one of a winged hymenopterous insects.*	mavu
water *A colorless, odorless liquid.*	maji
wax *Cerumen.*	nta ya sikio
weak *Feeble or deconditioned.*	dhaifu
weakness *Feebleness.*	udhaifu
weekly *That which occurs every seven days.*	kila wiki
weep, to *To ooze fluid, such as from a wound.*	vuja kwa maji kutoka jeraha
weep, to *To shed tears.*	kulia
wet *Covered in moisture.*	enye maji
wheal *A circumscribed urticarial lesion.*	kilengelenge rangi nyekundu
wheelchair *A wheeled device used for propulsion.*	gurudumu

English	Swahili
whisper *Speech in a volume that is barely discernible.*	mnong'ono
whistle, to *To make a high pitch noise by forcing air through the lips.*	mluzi
whitlow *An abscess occurring on the palmar surface of the fingertips.*	kaka
whooping cough *Pertussis*	kifaduro
widespread *Encompassing or spanning.*	kuenea
width *Side to side measurement.*	upana
wisdom tooth *Third molar.*	tatu cheyo
wise *Possessing much knowledge.*	busara
withdrawal *The action of being without drugs or alcohol.*	uondoaji
withhold, to *To refuse to give something.*	kuizuia
World Health Organization (WHO)	Shirika la Afya Duniani
worm *Any of long, slender, legless, soft-bodied invertebrates.*	mchango; mnyoo
worry, to *To fret or have unease.*	wasiwasi
worsen, to *To deteriorate.*	mbaya zaidi
wound *A tissue injury of varying severity.*	kidonda
wrist *The articulation of the hand and radius/ulna.*	kiwiko cha mkono; kilimbili
x-ray	uyoka; eksirei
xanthoma *A lipid deposition on the skin exhibited by an irregular yellow patch.*	doa njano kwenye ngozi
xerophthalmia *A manifestation of Vitamin A deficiency exhibited by dryness of the cornea and conjunctiva.*	Dalili za Upungufu wa vitamini A
xerosis *Pathological dryness of the skin or mucous membranes.*	ngozi kavu na utando wa kamasi
xiphoid process *The inferior segment of the sternum.*	sehemu ya chini ya mfupa wa kidari
yawn *Opening one's mouth and inhaling deeply due to sleepiness/boredom*	mwayo
yaws *A tropical disease characterized by ulcers on the extremities, caused by Treponema pertenue.*	buba
year *A time period that covers 365 days.*	mwaka
yearly *Occurring once each year.*	kila mwaka
yeast *A unicellular fungus.*	chachu
yell, to *To speak in a loud tone.*	piga kelele
yellow *A color between green and orange in the spectrum*	rangi ya manjano
yellow fever *A viral, hemorrhagic fever transmitted by mosquitos.*	homa ya manjano
young *Having lived for a short period.*	vijana
zero *No quantity.*	sifuri
zoology *The study of animals.*	utafiti wa wanyama
zoonosis *An animal-born disease that can be transmitted to humans, such as rabies.*	ugonjwa wa wanyama huambukizwa kwa binadamu
zymogen *An inactive compound that is metabolized to an active state.*	ugonjwa wa wanyama huambukizwa kwa binadamu

Swahili-English: A-kasumba

-a tumbo na msamba	**abdominoperineal** *Referring to the abdominal and perineal region.*
adha	**discomfort** *A feeling of physical or mental unease.*
adhifari	**perspiration from armpit (or bad body odor)**
adilifu	**fibrosis** *Connective tissue that is scarred and thickened after injury.*
afkani	**heart disease** *Generic term generally meant to imply coronary disease.*
afya	**health** *The state of being free of illness.*
aidha	**next** *The following or upcoming.*
aina damu	**blood type** *Determined and listed in the ABO system.*
aina ya bato	**favus** *Tinea capitis caused by Trichopyton schoenleini.*
aina ya damu	**ABO system** *The system using human blood antigens to determine blood type.*
aina ya damu	**blood grouping** *Testing blood to determine which type should be used for transfusion.*
aina ya minyoo ya tumbo	**ascaris** *A nematode from genus intestinal lumbricoid parasite, also called round worm.*
akili	**mental** *Cognitive or psychological.*
akimaanisha hisia za harufu	**olfactory** *Referring to the sense of smell.*
akimaanisha mapafu	**pulmonary** *Referring to the lungs.*
akimaanisha matiti	**mammary** *Referring to the breast.*
akimaanisha mfumo wa kusikia	**acoustic** *Referring to the auditory system.*
akimaanisha pua na koo	**nasopharyngeal** *Referring to the nose and pharynx.*
akimaanisha tishu wafu	**infarct** *Referring to dead tissue.*
akimaanisha usaha	**purulent** *Referring to pus.*
akimaanisha wakati kabla ya kuzaliwa	**prenatal** *Referring to the time prior to birth.*
akimaanisha ya njia ya haja kubwa	**rectal** *Referring to the rectum.*
akipiga sehemu ya uume; kichwa cha mboo	**glans penis** *The distal aspect of the penis.*
akrabu	**scorpion**
ala	**sheath** *A covering.*
ala ya kukombea	**curette** *The instrument used during a curettage.*
alfafa	**bandage tied to a circumcised penis**
ama mkono	**upper limb** *Referring to either arm.*
amelala	**asleep** *To be in a dormant or inactive state.*
asali	**syrup** *A thick sweet liquid.*
asidi	**acid** *Substance with a pH less than 7.*
asiye na meno	**toothless** *Edentulous.*
atika	**transplant,to** *To move a body part from one location to another.*
awali ya meno	**deciduous teeth** *The first teeth.*

-a tumbo na msamba	**abdominoperineal** *Referring to the abdominal and perineal region.*
baada ya ladha	**after-taste** *The sensation of a prolonged savor following eating/drinking.*
baadae ya matibabu tatizo kuhusiana na ugonjwa wa awali	**sequela** *A medical problem related to an initial injury or disease.(late sequelae)*
babaika	**stuttering** *Involuntary repetition of the first consonant.*
bakuli	**basin** *A small bowl used for washing.*
bandia	**artificial** *Not natural produced.*
bandia mwili sehemu	**prosthesis** *An artificial body part. (above the knee) [below the knee]*
bangi	**marijuana** *Cannabis.*
banzi	**brace** *A splint.*
baridi	**algid** *cold*
baridi	**cold** *Having a sense of being cold.*
baridi sana	**cold sore** *A perioral blister caused by herpes simplex.*
baridi yabisi	**rheumatism** *Any condition exhibited by inflammation and pain in the joints and muscles.*
bato	**tinea capitis** *Ringworm of the scalp, a fungal infection.*
bawasiri	**hemorrhoids** *Engorgement of the veins in the anus or rectum.*
bega	**shoulder** *The joint were the scapula joins the clavicle and humerus. (right shoulder, left shoulder)*
belghamu	**mucus** *A substance secreted by mucous membranes.*
belghamu kutoka pua	**rhinorrhea** *Abundant nasal mucosal drainage.*
bendeji	**bandage** *A strip of gauze used to immobilize or support.*
bendeji	**dressing** *The gauze applied to a wound.*
bendeji inatumika kuzuia kutokwa na damu	**pressure dressing** *A dressing used for compression to reduce bleeding.*
besofili	**basophil** *A polymorphonuclear granulocyte.*
bila fahamu	**unconsciousness** *Unable to respond to sensory stimuli.*
bila kuachilia yai	**anovulatory cycle** *A menstrual cycle in which no ovum is released.*
bila kujali	**regardless of** *Without consideration of.*
bila maumivu	**painless** *Not painful.*
bili	**bill** *A financial statement that indicates how much one owes.*
binadamu	**human** *Homo sapien.*
binti	**daughter**
biolojia	**biology** *The study of living organisms.*
boboka	**blurt out, to** *To speak without considering the repercussions.*
bombo	**influenza** *Viral infection causing fever, muscle aches and catarrh. (bombo also means pair of shorts in swahili)*
bonde la ufa homa	**Rift valley fever** *A human febrile illness that is an endemic disease in sheep, transmitted by mosquitos and direct contact and caused by a virus of the family Bunyaviridae.*
bora	**best** *Optimal or ideal.*
brachial mishipa ya fahamu	**brachial plexus** *A cluster of nerves coming off the last four cervical and first thoracic spinal nerves form the nerve supply the the chest and arms.*

-a tumbo na msamba	**abdominoperineal** *Referring to the abdominal and perineal region.*
buba	**framboesia; yaws** *An endemic tropical disease caused by Treponema pertenue.*
buba	**yaws** *A tropical disease characterized by ulcers on the extremities, caused by Treponema pertenue.*
bubu	**mute** *Refraining from or being speechless.*
bui	**tarantula** *A large hairy spider found mainly in the tropics.*
bumbauzi; (mshtuko)	**shock** *Surprise or astonishment. (startled)*
busara	**wise** *Possessing much knowledge.*
busha	**elephantiasis of the scrotum** *A condition caused by nematode parasites leading to lymphatic obstruction scrotal swelling.*
butu	**blunt** *Having a flat or rounded end.*
butu	**obtuse** *Rather insensitive or hard to understand.*
chachu	**sour** *An acid or bitter taste.*
chachu	**yeast** *A unicellular fungus.*
chafu	**dirty** *Unclean.*
chafu ya pus	**pyorrhea** *Emission of pus.*
chafuo; pange	**tsetse fly** *An insect that transmits the protozoa trypanosoma and can cause sleeping sickness.*
chakula	**food** *Nutrition.*
chakula bora	**nutrition** *The process of supplying food needed for growth.*
chakula sumu	**food poisoning** *Poisoning where the active agent is in the food.*
chale	**incision** *An intentional surgical cut in the skin.*
chale upasuaji wa figo	**nephrotomy** *Surgical incision of the kidney.*
chamko	**relapse** *The return to a prior state of ill health.*
chandalua	**mosquito net** *A fine mesh fabric hung over a bed as a mosquito repellent.*
chanjo	**immunization** *A medication given to provide immunity.*
chanjo	**inoculation** *Injection with a vaccine to provide immunity.*
chanjo	**vaccine** *A solution of attenuated microorganisms given to prevent or treat a disease.*
chanjo cheti	**vaccine certificate** *A document that denotes what vaccines have been received by the holder.*
chanjo ya kuzuia ungonjwa	**vaccination** *The act of receiving a vaccine.*
chanya	**positive** *Indicating the presence of something.*
chawa	**lice** *Plural for louse, a small parasite that lives on the skin. Pediculus humanus capitis is a head louse.*
chege	**genu varum** *A condition exhibited by the knees turning outward, commonly referred to as bowleg.*
chelewa	**late** *A time later than expected.*
cheti cha daktari	**prescription** *The action of prescribing a medication or treatment.*
chini	**down** *In a lower position.*
chini kiuno maumivu	**low back pain** *Pain in the lumbar region.*
chini kiuno maumivu	**lumbago** *Pain in the region of the lumbar spine.*
chini mdomo	**lip, lower** *Labium inferius oris.*
chini nyanja	**inferior** *The lower aspect.*
chini sana shinikizo la damu	**shock** *A condition characterized by systemic hypoperfusion.*

-a tumbo na msamba	**abdominoperineal** *Referring to the abdominal and perineal region.*
chini ya	**under; infra** *Sometimes used when indicating a patient is "under treatment" for a condition (active treatment).*
chini ya	**below** *Under.*
chini ya	**less** *A smaller amount.*
chini ya kucha za mikono au miguu	**subungual** *Under a fingernail or toenail.*
chini ya ngozi nyembamba ifunikayo ubongo na uti wa mgongo	**subdural** *The area between the dura mater and the arachnoid membrane.*
chini ya shinikizo la damu	**hypotension** *Abnormally low blood pressure.*
chini ya shinikizo la damu katika nafasi ya kusimama	**orthostatic** *Referring to the standing position. Orthostatic hypotension is low blood pressure in the standing position.*
chini ya taya	**submaxillary** *Situated below the maxilla.*
chini ya tumbo	**abdomen, lower**
chini ya ulimi	**sublingual** *Situated under the tongue.*
choa	**ringworm** *A fungal skin infection exhibited by pruritic well circumscribed patches on the scalp or feet.*
choa	**tinea** *Medical term for ringworm.*
choa ya kinena	**jock itch** *Pruritus caused by tinea cruris.*
choa ya kinena	**tinea cruris** *Ringworm in the inguinal region, a fungal infection.*
choa ya mwili	**tinea corporis** *Ringworm of the body, a fungal infection.*
choa ya uso	**tinea barbae** *Ringworm on the face in the region a man shaves.*
chokea	**hordeolum** *Inflammation of the sebaceous gland of the eye.*
chokea	**sty** *Also called hordeolum externum, it is inflammation of the sebaceous gland of an eyelash.*
choma	**burn** *An injury caused by exposure to heat.*
chomba cha kukojolea	**urinal** *Device used by men to void while in bed or sitting.*
chombo upasuaji kutumika kuvuta nyuma tishu	**retractor** *A device for pulling back tissue during surgery.*
chubua; kwaruza	**scrape** *An injury caused by having a body part rubbed against a rough surface.*
chubuko	**bruise** *Common term for ecchymosis.*
chubuko	**contusion** *An area of broken capillaries in the skin causing discoloration; commonly called a bruise.*
chuchu; titi	**nipple** *The small projection on the breast thru which milk is secreted.*
chuma kifaa kutumika kuwezesha kutembea	**walker** *A metal frame used to facilitate walking.*
chumba katika hospitali	**ward** *A section of a hospital where patients reside.*
chumvi	**salt** *Typically referring to sodium chloride.*
chumvi	**sodium chloride** *A colorless, crystalline compound; also table salt.*
chumvi	**salt** *Typically referring to sodium chloride.*
chungu	**bitter (taste)** *Having a harsh, unpleasant taste.*
chungu ya muda mrefu simika	**priapism** *A painful and abnormally prolonged erection.*
chunjua	**verruca** *A hyperplastic epidermal lesion, sometimes referred to as plantar wart.*

124

-a tumbo na msamba	**abdominoperineal** *Referring to the abdominal and perineal region.*
chunjua	**wart** *A flesh colored growth that is also called verruca.*
chunjua wa zinaa	**venereal wart** *Common term for condyloma acuminatum.*
chunjua ya wayo	**plantar wart** *A viral epidermal growth on the bottom of the foot.*
chunusi	**acne** *Inflamed or infected sebaceous glands.*
chupa	**bottle** *A container used for the storage of liquids.*
chupa	**flask** *A narrow-necked container.*
chura	**frog** *A tailless amphibian that is short with long hind legs for jumping.*
dakika	**minute** *Something very small.*
daktari kwa kutumia mikono yake bonyeza tumbo	**palpation** *The assessment of the body with the use of one's hands.*
daktari kwa upasuaji	**surgeon** *A physician who performs surgery.*
daktari wa kansa	**oncologist** *A physician specializing in the treatment of cancer.*
daktari wa macho	**ophthalmologist** *A physician specializing in diseases of the eye.*
daktari wa macho	**optometrist** *A person who practices optometry.*
daktari wa meno; tabibumeno; mhazigimeno	**dentist** *A professional capable of treating diseases of the teeth and gums.*
daktari wa mtoto	**pediatrician** *Physician who is a specialist in pediatrics.*
daktari; mganga	**physician** *Medical practitioner.*
dalili	**symptom** *A physical feature that is characteristic of disease.*
dalili awali	**presenting symptom** *The initial subjective complaint that initiated a visit.*
Dalili za Upungufu wa vitamini A	**xerophthalmia** *A manifestation of Vitamin A deficiency exhibited by dryness of the cornea and conjunctiva.*
damu	**blood** *Plasma containing erythrocytes, leukocytes and platelets.*
damu au mkojo sampuli	**specimen** *A sample for medical testing.*
damu chombo kwamba anarudi damu kutoka kwenye ubongo na moyo	**jugular vein (s)** *Includes the internal, external and anterior jugular veins.*
damu inapojikusanya pamoja	**hematoma** *A mass containing blood.*
damu kutoka mji wa mimba	**uterine bleeding** *Bleeding that emanates from the uterus.*
damu pombe ngazi	**blood alcohol level** *A quantitative measurement of the amount of alcohol in the blood.*
damu ya mwezi	**menses** *The blood and other material expelled from the uterus during menstruation.*
darubini ya uchunguzi wa mkojo	**urinalysis** *Chemical and microscopic examination of the urine.*
darubini; hadubini	**microscope** *A instrument used to magnify and view small objects.*
dawa	**drug** *A medication, sometimes with negative connotation.*
dawa ambayo hupunguza viwango vya sukari damu	**insulin** *A hormone produced by the pancreas and synthetically to control blood glucose levels.*
dawa ambayo kuharibu minyoo ya tumbo	**ascaricide** *Agent that destroys ascaris.*
dawa kufutwa katika kioevu	**elixir** *A medical solution.*

-a tumbo na msamba	**abdominoperineal** *Referring to the abdominal and perineal region.*
dawa kuharibu minyoo ya tumbo	**anthelmintic** *An agent used to destroy worms.*
dawa kutolewa katika mkundu au uke	**suppository** *A delivery system for medication placed in an orifice.*
dawa kutumika kukabiliana na sumu; kiuasumu	**antidote** *A medication that neutralizes a toxin.*
dawa kutumika kuondoa maumivu	**analgesic** *A medication used to remove pain.*
dawa kutumika kupunguza kikohozi	**antitussive** *Medication used to diminish a cough.*
dawa kutumika kupunguza uvimbe	**anti-inflammatory** *Medication used to reduce inflammation.*
dawa kutumika kutibu huzuni	**antidepressant** *Medication used to treat depression.*
dawa kutumika kutibu kifafa	**anticonvulsant** *Medication used to treat seizures.*
dawa kutumika kutibu kuwasha	**antipruritic** *Medication used to treat pruritus.*
dawa kutumika kutibu malaria	**antimalarial** *Medication used to treat malaria.*
dawa kutumika kutibu maumivu ya kichwa	**antimigraine** *Medication used to treat headaches.*
dawa kutumika kutibu vya magonjwa	**antibiotic** *A medication that inhibits or kills microorganisms.*
dawa kutumika kwa ajili ya tulizo	**sedative** *A medication used to facilitate sleep or calm a person.*
dawa kutumika kwa kupunguza wasiwasi	**tranquilizer** *A medication used to diminish anxiety.*
dawa kutumika nyembamba ya damu	**anticoagulant** *Medication used to inhibit coagulation.*
dawa makao marashi	**ointment** *A petroleum jelly based topical medication.*
dawa ya kuharibu nguvu ya sumu ya nyoka	**antivenin** *An antitoxin formulated for various types of snake bites.*
dawa ya kuondoa au kuua viini vya magonjwa	**disinfectant** *A substance that kills bacteria.*
dawa ya makuru kutumika kulainisha ngozi au kupunguza maumivu	**emollient** *Having softening or soothing qualities.*
dawa zinazotumika kutibu homa	**antipyretic** *Medication used to treat fever.*
dhahabu	**gold** *Precious metal with atomic number of 79.*
dhahiri	**evident** *Obvious.*
dhaifu	**weak** *Feeble or deconditioned.*
dhaifu na kizunguzungu	**faint** *Weak and dizzy.*
dharura	**emergency** *An urgent, life-threatening situation.*
dharura chumba	**emergency room** *A ward used for initial treatment of critical patients.*
dhiki	**anguish** *Significant mental or physical pain.*
dhiki; ugonjwa sifa kwa wazimu, mtazamo udanganyifu, kuharibika	**schizophrenia** *A chronic mental condition exhibited by delusions, hallucinations, and faulty perception.*
doa	**blemish** *A small mark on one's skin.*
doa ngozini	**macula solaris** *Formal medical term describing a freckle.*

126

-a tumbo na msamba	**abdominoperineal** *Referring to the abdominal and perineal region.*
doa njano kwenye ngozi	**xanthoma** *A lipid deposition on the skin exhibited by an irregular yellow patch.*
dogo	**trivial** *Of little importance or value.*
donda	**ulcer** *A concave wound caused by a break in the integrity of skin or mucous membrane. (duodenal ulcer)*
donda kidonda	**canker sore** *An ulceration, usually of the mouth or lips.*
dondakoo	**diphtheria** *A contagious bacterial disease characterized by a grey membrane on the pharynx along with respiratory or cutaneous symptoms; caused by Corynebacterium diphtheriae.*
donge la damu	**blood clot** *A mass of coagulated blood.*
duka la madawa	**pharmacy** *A business that sells prescription medication.*
dunga jeraha	**stab wound** *An injury occurring with a sharp object.*
duta	**rebound** *A term used to describe a type of tenderness found with peritonitis.*
Dutu hii ambayo inaweza kusababisha mmenyuko mzio	**allergen** *Compound that causes an allergic reaction.*
elimu	**education** *Instruction or guidance.*
elimu ya mawazo	**psychology** *The study of the human mind and emotions.*
embamba	**thin** *Lean or slender.*
enda choo; enda mavi	**defecation** *The discharge of feces from the rectum.*
endeleo	**growth** *The increase in physical size.*
eneo dogo la uvimbe	**puffiness** *Having a soft, swollen area.*
eneo la kifua kati ya mapafu	**mediastinum** *The thoracic area between the lungs.*
enye maji	**wet** *Covered in moisture.*
enye mishipa ya damu	**vascular** *Referring to a blood vessel.*
epesi	**light** *Not heavy.*
erisipela	**erysipelas** *An acute infection caused by Streptococcus pyogenes that causes fever along with swelling and inflammation. The infection frequently effects the face or one leg.*
fadhaa	**agitation** *A state of extreme emotional disturbance.*
familia	**family**
fanya kuwa sabuni	**saponify,to** *The creation of soap from oil using an alkali.*
feri	**iron** *An element found in hemoglobin.*
feri upungufu safura	**iron-deficiency anemia** *A microcytic anemia.*
fidhuli	**rude** *Ill-mannered.*
figo; buki	**kidney** *One of two glandular organs that form urine.*
firigisi-firigisi	**craw-craw** *A pruritic papular skin eruption sometimes caused by Onchocerca.*
fuama	**knee elbow position** *Knees and elbows are on the table and the chest is in the air.*
fudifudi; uso chini	**prone** *Lying with the abdomen and face downward.*
funda	**mouthful** *A large quantity of something in one's mouth.*
fundo	**knot** *A fastening made by tying a suture, for instance.*
funga choo	**constipation** *A condition exhibited by difficulty in having a bowel movement due to hard stools.*
fuzi	**acromioclavicular joint** *Referring to the junction of the acromion and clavicle. (shoulder)*

-a tumbo na msamba	**abdominoperineal** *Referring to the abdominal and perineal region.*
fyonza	**suck, to** *As in, to suction fluid.*
gaagaa	**restless, to be** *Wriggle or squirm. Extreme restlessness, tossing around in bed.*
gango	**splint** *A rigid support used to immobilize and extremity.*
ganzi	**numbness** *Decreased sensation to tactile stimuli.*
ganzi	**paresthesia** *An abnormal sensation usually described as pins and needles.*
ganzi; nusukaputi	**anesthesia** *Loss of sensation.*
gari kwamba hubeba wagonjwa au kujeruhiwa	**ambulance** *A vehicle that carries the sick or injured.*
gegedu	**cartilage** *Firm, relatively non-vascular connective tissue.*
gego	**molar tooth** *Any of the most posterior teeth bilaterally which includes 8 deciduous and usually 12 permanent teeth.*
ghadhabu	**rage** *Uncontrollable anger.*
ghafla	**abrupt** *Suddenly or hastily.*
ghafla kupoteza fahamu	**syncope** *Sudden loss of consciousness.*
ghafla mbaya	**flare-up** *A sudden worsening one's condition.*
ghamu; soda	**depressed** *Melancholy.*
gharama	**cost** *The fee or penalty.*
glakoma	**glaucoma** *A condition characterized by increased intraocular pressure.*
glascow kukosa fahamu wadogo	**Glasgow coma scale** *A scale used to grade one's level of consciousness with a score of 3 being totally unresponsive and a score of 15 being normal.*
glavu	**gloves** *Covering for hand protection.*
goigoi	**indolent** *1. Causing little pain. 2. Slow healing ulcer.*
gonjwa	**pandemic** *When a disease is present over an entire region.*
gorofa	**flat** *Level or even; without bulges.*
gorofa mvungo wa wayo	**pes planus** *Medical term for flat foot.*
gorofa-mguu	**flatfoot** *Common term for pes planus.*
goti	**knee** *The joint at the distal femur and proximal tibia.*
govi; zunga	**foreskin** *Also called prepuce, the skin that naturally covers the glans but can be rolled back.*
Guinea ya mdudu	**guinea worm** *A parasitic nematode worm that, in cases of infection, lives under the skin, formally called Dracunculus medinensis.*
gumu	**induration** *An area that is abnormally hard.*
gundi	**glue** *Plastic cements*
gurudumu	**wheelchair** *A wheeled device used for propulsion.*
gusa	**touch** *Tactile stimulation.*
gutu la mguu au mkono	**stump** *Term used to designate what remains of an amputated extremity.*
hadhi ya ndoa	**marital status** *Single versus married status.*
hafifu	**benign** *Not harmful.*
haijulikani	**unknown** *Uncertain or undisclosed.*
haitoshi damu ugavi	**ischemia** *Inadequate blood supply to a part of the body.*
haja	**need** *A want or obligation.*

128

-a tumbo na msamba	**abdominoperineal** *Referring to the abdominal and perineal region.*
haki	**fair** *Equitable.*
haki	**right** *Justice or fairness.(noun)*
hakuna mtiririko wa damu na sehemu ya kuoza mwili na ya baadae ya sehemu ambayo	**necrosis** *The death of most of the cells of the affected part.*
hali	**inertia** *The tendency to remain unchanged.*
hali ambapo kichwa cha mgonjwa huinuliwa juu ya moyo hasa kwa kusaidia kutibu kuzilai	**trendelenburg position** *Position in bed in which the head is lower than the feet.*
hali ambapo sehemu iliyo kati ya moyo na ngozi inzungukao moyo hujazwa na maji ya mwili	**pericardial tamponade** *Decrease in systemic perfusion related to a collection of fluid in the pericardial space.*
hali ambapo vena ya shingo hupanuka	**jugular venous distension** *Enlarged jugular veins caused by high pulmonary capillary pressure.*
hali inayoletwa na kuongezeka kwa viini au sumu kwenye damu	**sepsis** *A condition exhibited by overwhelming inflammation due to infection.*
hali inayoletwa na kupungua kwa asidi mwilini	**alkalosis** *A condition in which the pH is increased.*
hali isiyo ya kawaida chini joto la mwili	**hypothermia** *Lower than normal temperature.*
hali isiyo ya kawaida kiasi kidogo cha damu ya hedhi	**oligomenorrhea** *Infrequent menstruation or low volume menstrual flow.*
hali isiyo ya kawaida kichwa ndogo	**microcephalic** *A congenital deformity exhibited by an abnormally small head.*
hali isiyo ya kawaida kubwa kiasi cha damu ya hedhi	**menorrhagia** *Abnormally large amount of menstrual blood.*
hali isiyo ya kawaida kubwa kichwa	**macroencephaly** *Having an abnormally large head.*
hali isiyo ya kawaida kubwa midomo	**macrocheilia** *Abnormally large lips.*
hali isiyo ya kawaida kubwa ulimi	**macroglossia** *Abnormally large tongue.*
hali isiyo ya kawaida kubwa vidole	**macrodactyly** *Abnormally large digits.*
hali isiyo ya kawaida ndogo kiasi cha nywele mwili	**oligotrophia or hypotrichosis** *Less than normal amount of head/body hair.*
hali isiyo ya kawaida ndogo kiasi cha pato mkojo	**oliguria** *Abnormally low urine output.*
hali isiyo ya kawaida ndogo taya	**micrognathia** *Abnormally small maxilla or mandible.*
hali isiyo ya kawaida nene ngozi	**pachydermia** *An abnormally thick skin.*
hali isiyo ya kawaida nyembamba na dhaifu	**emaciation** *Abnormally thin and weak.*
hali isiyo ya kawaida ya juu mvungo wa wayo	**pes cavus** *Excessive height of the longitudinal arch of the foot.*

-a tumbo na msamba	**abdominoperineal** *Referring to the abdominal and perineal region.*
hali ya arteri kupata ugumu, kusongana na kupoteza uwezo wa kunyumbuka au kurefuka	**arteriosclerosis** *Hardening and thickening of arterial walls.*
hali ya kikohozi gumio	**croup** *An acute laryngeal condition that is accompanied by a hoarse, barking cough*
hali ya kupoteza uguma wa mifupa	**osteoporosis** *Loss of bone substance because the osteoblasts fail to produce bone matrix.*
hali ya kupungua kwa sukari kwenye damu	**hypoglycemia** *Abnormally low blood sugar.*
hali ya kuwa na chawa	**pediculosis** *Lice infestation.*
hali ya kuzimia roho	**coma** *A state of unconsciousness.*
hali ya mtoto kutangulia na matako anapozaliwa	**breech presentation** *Position of the feet or buttocks near the cervix.*
hali ya mtoto kutangulia na uso anapozaliwa	**face presentation** *Referring to the part of the body coming out of the cervix first during childbirth.*
hali ya ngozi na sifa ya malengelenge kubwa	**pemphigus** *A skin disorder with large bullous lesions.*
hali ya sifa na kichwa kuwa akageuka katika mwelekeo mmoja kuendelea	**torticollis** *A condition exhibited by the head being turned to one side continuously.*
halula	**peritonsillar abscess**
hamu kubwa ya kupumua lakini kutokuwa na uwezo	**air hunger** *The sensation of shortness of breath.*
hamu ya chakula	**appetite** *A desire to eat.*
haraka jicho harakati	**Rapid Eye Movement** *The movement of a person's eyes during this period of sleep.*
haraka jicho harakati wakati wa kulala	**REM (rapid eye movement) sleep** *This period of sleep is associated with irregular respirations and heart rate, involuntary movements and dreaming.*
haraka mwendo usio wa hiari ya macho	**nystagmus** *Rapid involuntary movement of the eyes; it can be horizontal, vertical or rotary.*
harara	**prickly heat** *A rash with small vesicles that is pruritic and associated with a warm moist environment. Also called miliaria rubra.*
harisho	**diarrhea** *Increase in frequency and a loose consistency of the stools.*
harufu	**odor** *A smell that is given off someone or something.*
hataki	**negative** *Contrary or opposing.*
hatari	**malignant** *Tendency of a tumor to invade normal tissue.*
hatua	**milestone** *An event indicative of a certain stage of development.*
hawajui kusoma na kuandika	**illiterate** *Unable to read or write.*
haya usoni	**blush, to** *To have an increased volume of blood flow to one's face causing a red tint to the skin.*
hewa	**air**
hiari	**elective** *Non-urgent and not life-saving.*
hima	**brisk** *Rapid or fast.*
hisia	**emotion** *An intense feeling.*
hivyo	**hence** *Thus.*
hofu	**fear** *Fright or trepidation.*

-a tumbo na msamba	**abdominoperineal** *Referring to the abdominal and perineal region.*
hofu kubwa ya kitu	**phobia** *An profound fear of something.*
homa	**febrile** *Presence of an supraphysiologic temperature.*
homa	**fever** *A temperature above the normal range.*
homa	**hyperpyrexia** *Fever.*
homa	**hyperthermia** *Fever.*
homa	**pyrexia** *Fever.*
homa iletwayo na usubi	**sandfly fever** *A febrile illness transmitted by a sandfly, from the genus Phlebotomus, and found in the Mediterranean.*
homa iletwayo na usubi	**sandfly fever** *A febrile illness transmitted by a sandfly, from the genus Phlebotomus, and found in the Mediterranean.*
homa kiwimbi	**undulant fever** *Wave-like variations in the fever, going from very high to normal and back again, as seen in Brucellosis.*
homa na kutetemeka; kitapo	**ague** *A term used to describe recurrent fever and shivering typically associated with malaria.*
homa ya manjano	**icterus** *Yellowing of the skin and sclerae because of excess bilirubin.*
homa ya manjano	**jaundice** *Yellowing of the sclerae and skin because of excessive bilirubin in the blood.*
homa ya manjano	**yellow fever** *A viral, hemorrhagic fever transmitted by mosquitos.*
homa ya manjano ya mtoto mchanga	**jaundice of the newborn** *A form of jaundice seen in newborns in the first two weeks of life; also called icterus neonatorum.*
homa ya matumbo	**typhoid fever** *A condition caused by ingestion of food or water containing salmonella typhi that is exhibited by fever and abdominal signs and symptoms.*
homa ya mbu; malaria	**malaria** *A condition caused by a protozoan of the genus Plasmodium. It is transmitted by mosquitos and is exhibited by fever, chills, headache. In the severe form it can lead to convulsions, increased ICP and death.*
homa ya papasi	**tick-borne fever** *A relapsing fever caused by a spirochete of the genus Borrelia.*
homa ya vipele vyekundu	**scarlet fever** *A condition caused by streptococci that is exhibited by fever and a bright red (scarlet) rash.*
hospitali	**hospital** *Acute care medical/surgical facility.*
huduma	**assistance** *The act of helping.*
huduma ya kwanza	**first aid** *The initial treatment after an injury.*
huduma ya matibabu ya wazee	**geriatrics** *The study of the health of old people.*
hulisonga	**choke** *To retch, cough or fight for breath.*
huntha	**hermaphrodite** *A person possessing gonadal characteristics of both sexes.*
huweza kuingia	**impervious** *Not affected by.*
huzuni	**grief** *Deep sorrow.*
idhini	**approval** *Accepting something as satisfactory.*
ikiwa na mgongo	**scoliosis** *A lateral curvature of the spine.*
ikiwa utoaji mimba	**induced abortion** *Surgical or medical evacuation of the fetus.*
ila	**defect** *A shortcoming or imperfection.*

-a tumbo na msamba	**abdominoperineal** *Referring to the abdominal and perineal region.*
ile ngozi ya katikati kabisa kati ya zile tatu zizungukazo ubongo na uti wa mgongo	**subarachnoid** *The layer of the brain covering between the arachnoid and pia mater.*
iliongezeka sukari katika damu	**hyperglycemia** *Higher than normal level of glucose in the blood.*
ilipungua ngozi unyeti	**hypoesthesia** *Abnormally decreased skin sensitivity.*
imara	**firm** *Hard or unyielding.*
imara	**stamina** *Ability to maintain physical or mental exertion for a long period.*
imara kupotoka ya gumba	**hallux valgus** *Also called bunion, it is the lateral deviation of the great toe.*
inao uhusiano na machozi	**lacrimal** *Referring to the secretion of tears.*
inapatikana	**available** *Attainable, obtainable.*
inatisha ndoto	**nightmare** *An unpleasant or frightening dream.*
inayoendelea	**on going** *Continuing,*
inayohusiana na mifupa mifupi na mipana ya mkono sehemu ya chini	**radial** *Referring to the radius.*
inayohusiana na moyo, mishipa ya damu na damu	**cardiovascular** *Referring to the heart or circulatory system.*
inayojulikana	**known** *Recognized or familiar.*
inayojulikana lakini isiyopaswa madhara ya dawa	**side effect** *An expected but unwanted effect of a medication.*
inayotokea pole pole, huchukua muda mrefu, isiyo ya ghafla	**chronic** *When referring to an illness, it means recurring or persistent.*
ini	**liver** *A large glandular organ in the right upper quadrant that functions in digestive processes, as well as, neutralizing toxins.*
ini jipu	**liver abscess** *A localized collection of pus in the liver.*
ishara ya hofu	**panic attack** *Sudden, profound anxiety.*
ishara za kuonyesha kuwa wakati wa damu ya kila mwezi umekaribia	**premenstrual syndrome** *A cluster of emotional, behavioral, and physical symptoms that occur in the premenstrual phase of the menstrual cycle and resolve with the onset of menstruation.*
isiyo ya kawaida na kumbukumbu nzuri	**hypermnesia** *Unusually good memory.*
istiska	**ascites** *Serous fluid in the abdominal cavity.*
itakayosaidia	**adjuvant** *Term used to describe the medical treatment after initial therapy, as in adjuvant radiation therapy after initial chemotherapy.*
jamidi	**frostbite** *Local tissue destruction after exposure to cold.*
jansi ya uso vinavyosababisha moja upande mmoja tabasamu	**risus sardonicus** *A spasm of the facial muscles causing what appears to be a smile on one's face.*
jaribio la pumzi kwa ajili ya pombe	**breath test (for alcohol)** *A check of alcohol level by testing exhaled air.*
jasho mengi	**diaphoretic** *Exhibited by profuse perspiration.*
jasho; hari	**sweat** *Moisture exuded through the pores of the skin.*
jeni	**gene** *A unit of heredity that is passed on from parent to child.*

-a tumbo na msamba	**abdominoperineal** *Referring to the abdominal and perineal region.*
jeraha la baridi ambalo sio la kuganda ambalo huletwa na baridi au majimaji hali inayozuia damu kutembea vizuri	**immersion foot** *After prolonged cold exposure the foot is cold and numb. As it rewarms, it becomes hyperemic, paresthetic and hyperhidrotic.*
jicho matone	**eye drops** *Liquid applied to eyes for various medical problems.*
jina	**name** *A word by which a person is known.*
jina	**surname** *One's given "last" name that generally changes for women upon marriage to that of the man's surname.*
jino	**tooth** *One of a set of hard, bony enamel coated structure in the jaw.*
jino chongo	**canine teeth** *Located between the incisors and premolars.*
jino la mbele	**incisor** *Sharp-edged tooth; humans have four incisors.*
jinsia	**sex** *Gender.*
jipu	**furuncle** *A painful erythematous nodule with a central core.*
jipu	**boil** *Small abscess or furuncle.*
jipu (majipu)	**abscess** *A localized collection of pus.*
jipu kwenye ufizi	**gumboil** *Swelling noted on the gingiva over a dental abscess.*
jipu la kifuko au kiwasho	**quinsy** *Peritonsillar inflammation or abscess.*
jipu la mtoki	**bubo** *An inflamed, swollen lymph node in the axilla or inguinal region.*
jipu ya uti wa mgongo	**spinal cord abscess** *A localized collection of purulent material in or adjacent to the spinal cord.*
jirani figo	**perinephric** *Around the kidney.*
jisua	**gag** *Choke or retch.*
jongo	**gout** *Monosodium urate crystal deposition disease.*
joto	**heat** *The quality of being hot.*
joto kiharusi	**heat stroke** *A condition caused by excessive exposure to high ambient temperature; it is exhibited by dry skin, thirst, vertigo, muscle cramps and nausea. The three forms are heat exhaustion, heat cramps and sunstroke.*
juhudi	**effort** *Attempt or endeavor.*
juu	**high** *Elevated.*
juu	**superior** *In a position above something else.*
juu mdomo	**lip, upper** *Labium superius oris.*
juu ya wayo (mguuni) pahali moyo husikika ukipiga	**dorsalis pedis pulse** *Pulse on dorsum of the foot.*
juu, juu ya	**above**
kaa chawa	**crab louse** *Phthirus pubis is formal name for a louse that infests pubic hair and causes intense itching.*
kaakaa	**palate** *The roof of the mouth.*
kabisa	**absolute**
kabla ya	**beforehand** *In advance or previously.*
kabla ya kuanza kwa hedhi	**premenstrual** *Occurring prior to the onset of menstruation.*
kaka	**whitlow** *An abscess occurring on the palmar surface of the fingertips.*

133

-a tumbo na msamba	**abdominoperineal** *Referring to the abdominal and perineal region.*
kalab	**rabies** *An infectious viral disease transmitted through the bite of a mammal. Symptoms include hydrophobia, pharyngeal spasms and hyperactivity.*
kali	**mild** *Slight, nominal.*
kali	**severe** *Intense or very great.*
kali kiasi	**subacute** *A stage between acute and chronic.*
kali kukonda	**cachexia** *Generalized weakness and severe wasting.*
kalsiamu	**calcium** *A chemical element that is an essential component in teeth and bone.*
kama nywele	**cilia** *The hairs growing on the eyelid or a motile extension of a cell surface.*
kama uzi	**filiform** *Threadlike.*
kamasi	**nasal mucus** *Secretions coming from the nose.*
kamata; mkamba	**pneumonia** *Inflammation of the lung due to an infection caused by a virus or bacterium.*
kamwe kupewa kuzaliwa	**nullipara** *A woman who has never given birth.*
kamwe kuwa mjamzito	**nulligravida** *A woman who has never been pregnant.*
kang'ata	**rheumatic pain** *Pain related to rheumatoid arthritis.*
kansa; saratani	**cancer; carcinoma** *A disease of uncontrolled abnormal cell growth.*
Kaposis sarcoma	**Kaposi sarcoma** *Typically seen in AIDS patients, it is characterized by cutaneous reddish-purple macules and plaques.Also called multiple idiopathic hemorrhagic sarcoma.*
karantini	**quarantine** *A place of isolation for infectious persons until it can be certain it is safe to let them mingle.*
karibu	**around** *On every side of.*
karibu	**near** *In close proximity.*
karibu kifu	**moribund** *Near death.*
karibu na kiungo	**juxta-articular** *Positioned near a joint.*
karibu na mjiko	**pararectal** *Adjacent to the rectum.*
karibu na mwisho	**end stage** *Terminal stage. End stage cancer means there is no cure possible and death is imminent.*
karibu na pua	**paranasal** *Situated adjacent to the nose.*
kasi	**pace** *Consistent and continuous movement.*
kasiba ya kukaa katika kibofu cha mkojo mkojo	**indwelling catheter** *Continuous use tube usually referring to a tube in the urinary bladder.*
kasumba	**opium** *An addictive drug derived from opium poppy; synthetic versions are used as analgesics.*
-a tumbo na msamba	**abdominoperineal** *Referring to the abdominal and perineal region.*

Swahili-English: kaswende-kuondoa nguo

Swahili	English
kaswende; sekeneko	**syphilis** *A infectious disease caused by Treponema pallidum that causes a painless penile ulcer in the primary stage but can lead to irreversible brain damage in the untreated tertiary stage.*
kati	**center** *A point equidistant from all sides.*
katika mfululizo	**serial** *In a series.*
katikati ; karibu na katikati	**medial** *Situated toward the midline.*
katikati ya mbavu	**intercostal** *Area between the ribs*
katikati ya sikio	**ear, middle** *Auris media.*
kavu	**dry** *Absence of moisture.*
kavu kikohozi	**dry cough** *A cough without sputum production.*
kavu rishai	**crust** *Dried serous exudate covering a wound.*
kavu, ngumu, wafu tishu	**eschar** *Dry, hard, dead tissue commonly seen with a chronic pressure ulcer or anthrax.*
kawaida	**common** *That which is usual.*
kawaida	**usual** *Typical or normal.*
kawaida kiasi cha hedhi lakini katika vipindi kawaida	**metrorrhagia** *Uterine bleeding in normal amounts but at irregular intervals.*
kekee	**drill** *Cylindrical metal tool uses for creating a hole in bone in surgery.*
kemikali cha uwezo wa kuua manii	**spermicide** *A substance capable of killing sperm.*
kemotaksi	**chemotaxis** *The response of an organism to chemical agents.*
kengeza	**squint, to** *To look at something with the eyes partially closed.*
kiamo	**colostrum** *The fluid secreted by the mammary glands a few days around parturition.*
kiasi	**amount** *The total or the aggregate.*
kiasi cha hewa ambacho mtu anapumua mara moja anapovuta pumzi katika hali ya kuwaida	**tidal volume** *The amount of air inspired with each breath. One can set a ventilator to deliver a preset number of milliliters of oxygenated air with each breath.*
kiasi kidogo ya maji yanayozunguka kijusi	**oligohydramnios** *Inadequate amount of amniotic fluid.*
kiasili	**indigenous** *Naturally occurring.*
kiatu	**shoe** *Article of clothing worn on each foot.*
kibali	**clearance** *The process of removing something.*
kibanzi	**splinter** *A small, thin object; usually refers to the object being imbedded in the body.*
kibeti; kibushuti	**dwarf** *Abnormally small person.*
kibofu cha mkojo	**bladder, urinary** *Vestibule for urine prior to being expelled via the urethra.*
kibofu cha mkojo	**urinary bladder** *The organ collecting urine from the ureters prior to discharge via the urethra.*
kibofu cha nyongo	**gallbladder** *The organ adjacent to the liver that stores bile and secretes it into the duodenum.*

Swahili	English
kibogoyo	**toothless person**
kibole	**appendix** *An appendage of the cecum.*
kiboleini	**hydrocele** *The accumulation of fluid in a body sac.*
kichaa; wazimu	**insanity** *Referring to a serious mental illness.*
kichanga ngiri	**exomphalos** *Umbilical hernia*
kichanga ngiri	**hernia, umbilical** *Protrusion of abdominal contents at the umbilicus.*
kichefuchefu	**nausea** *A feeling that one wants to vomit.*
kichocho	**Bilharzia** *Historical name of a genus of flukes or nematodes now known as Schistosoma.*
kichocho	**schistosomiasis** *A condition, sometimes known as bilharzia, which involves infestation with flukes of the genus Schistosoma.*
kichomi	**stabbing pain** *A sharp piercing quality to pain.*
kichomi ya tumbo	**stomach cramps** *Sensation of muscle contraction in the epigastric area.*
kichwa	**caput** *The head.*
kichwa	**head**
kichwani	**scalp** *The skin covering the head except for the face.*
kidaka tonge	**epiglottis** *Tissue at the base of the tongue that covers the trachea when one swallows.*
kidaka tonge; kimio	**uvula** *A fleshy pendent at the back of the soft palate.*
kidevu	**chin** *Mentum; the anterior projection of the lower jaw.*
kidogo	**slight** *Minor or small.*
kidogo kidogo	**drop by drop** *Expression meaning little by little.*
kidole	**digit** *Finger.*
kidole cha mguu	**toe** *Any of the digits of of the feet.*
kidole cha mkono	**finger** *Any of the five digits on the hand.*
kidole gumba	**thumb** *The first digit of each hand.*
kidole kwa muda mrefu mwembamba	**arachnodactyly** *A condition exhibited by abnormally long and slender fingers.*
kidoletumbo	**appendicitis** *Inflammation of the appendix.*
kidonda	**wound** *A tissue injury of varying severity.*
kidonda katika mfuko wa tumbo na chango	**gastroduodenal ulcer** *A lesion in the mucosal lining of the stomach or duodenum.*
kidonda kutoka kuwekewa gorofa katika kitanda	**decubitus ulcer** *A wound caused by laying in one position for too long; also referred to as a pressure ulcer.*
kidonda kuwa matokeo kutoka kuwekewa kitandani kwa muda wa siku nyingi	**pressure ulcer** *Loss in skin integrity due to a portion of the body being in the same position for too long and possibly other factors.*
kidusia vinavyosababisha maambukizi ya upungufu wa damu	**hookworm** *A parasitic infection of the family Strongylidae that can cause anemia.*
kidutu	**comedone** *The medical term (singular) for blackheads.*
kifaa kama mrija kinachotiwa mwilini ili kutoa au kutia vitu vya aina ya majimaji	**catheter** *A flexible tube inserted into the body.*
kifaa kutumika kuomba dawa	**applicator** *A device used to apply a topical medication.*
kifaa kutumika kushikilia sindano	**needle holder** *A surgical instrument used to grasp a needle during suturing.*

Swahili	English
kifaa kutumika kutoa msaada kwa ajili ya ngiri	**truss** *A synthetic device for containing a hernia within the abdomen.*
kifaa kutumika kwa artificially kupumua kwa mgonjwa	**respirator** *A device used to artificially ventilate a patient.*
kifaa kwa kupima	**tape measure** *A long length of tape, marked at intervals for measuring.*
kifaa kwamba mabadiliko ya dawa kioevu katika ukungu kwa kuvuta pumzi	**nebulizer** *A device used for transforming a liquid into a fine mist for inhalation as in nebulized albuterol for an acute exacerbation of asthma.*
kifaduro	**pertussis** *Synonym for whooping cough.*
kifaduro	**whooping cough** *Pertussis*
kifafa	**epilepsy** *A condition associated with abnormal brain activity and exhibited by sudden, recurrent convulsions, sensory disturbances and loss of consciousness.*
kifafa mshtuko	**epileptic seizure** *A convulsion related to abnormal brain activity (as opposed to being precipitated by hypoglycemia.)*
kifafa mshtuko	**seizure** *An episode of tonic/clonic movement noted in epilepsy.*
kifafa na shinikizo la damu wakati wa ujauzito	**eclampsia** *A maternal condition characterized by convulsions and hypertension that can lead to maternal and fetal death.*
kifandugu	**coccyx** *The small bone formed by the natural fusion of rudimentary vertebrae.*
kifua	**thorax** *The part of the body between the neck and abdomen.*
kifua	**chest** *Thorax.*
kifua kikuu	**tuberculosis** *Any infectious disease caused by Mycobacterium.*
kifua maumivu yanayosababishwa na mtiririko maskini damu	**angina pectoris** *Exercise induced myocardial ischemia.*
kifua maumivu yanayosababishwa na mtiririko maskini damu	**anisomelia** *Unequal size of arms or legs.*
kifua ukuta	**chest wall** *Thoracic wall.*
kifuko cha moyoni; upande wa chini wa kila nusu ya moyo	**ventricle** *1. One of two chambers of the heart. 2. The four interconnected cavities in the center of the brain.*
kifuko pahali ambapo mayai hutengenezewa ndani ya tumbo la mwanamke	**ovary** *One of a paired of female reproductive glands containing oocytes.*
kifundo cha mguu	**ankle** *The area of the ankle joint.*
kifundo cha mguu uvimbe	**ankle swelling** *Enlargement of the ankle region with or without pitting.*
kifundo cha mguu wa mapafu	**ankle edema or dependent edema** *Extracellular fluid volume noted by swelling or pitting.*
kifundo cha mguu wa pamoja	**ankle joint** *The articulation of the tibia/fibula and talus.*
kifundo; kinundu	**nodule** *A small node in the skin of up to 1cm and in the lung up to 3cm.*
kifungo	**confinement** *As in confined to bed.*
kifuniko cha uso kinachozuia hewa kutoka	**non-rebreather mask** *A type of oxygen mask used to deliver a higher oxygen concentration.*
kigasha	**forearm** *Segment of the arm from the elbow to wrist.*
kigego	**abnormal**
kigongo	**hunchback** *Synonym of kyphosis.*

Swahili	English
kigongo	**kyphosis** *Abnormal outward curvature of the spine.*
kigosho cha miguu; yangekuwa goti	**genu valgum** *A condition exhibited by the knees turning inward, commonly referred to as knock-knee.*
kigosho cha miguu; yangekuwa goti	**knock knees** *Common term for genu valgum.*
kigugumizi	**stammer,to** *The impulse to repeat the first letter of words and involuntary pauses while speaking.*
kiguu	**talipes equinovaro** *Medical term for what is commonly known as club foot.*
kihafidhina	**conservative** *Control rather than elimination of a disease.*
kiharusi	**apoplexy** *Extravasation of blood within an organ. For example, neonatal apoplexy is consistent with intracranial hemorrhage.*
kiharusi	**poliomyelitis** *An infectious viral disease exhibited by constitutional symptoms that can lead to quadriplegia.*
kiharusi	**spasm** *An involuntary contraction of muscles.*
kiharusi	**stroke** *Common term for cerebrovascular accident.*
kiherehere cha moyo	**palpitation** *Sensation of a forceful, rapid, irregular heartbeat present after exercise or with anxiety.*
kiini cha jicho	**pupil** *The opening at the center of the iris.*
kiini chenye vitu kama nyuzi kipatikanacho kwenye maji ya juu	**giardiasis** *A flagellate protozoa, Giardia lamblia, that causes diarrhea.*
kiinitete	**embryo** *The term used to describe a fertilized ovum in the first 8 weeks of development.*
kijembe	**lancet** *A small sharp instrument used to obtain a drop of blood for testing.*
kijerumani surua	**German measles** *(rubella) A contagious viral infection.*
kijidudu	**germ** *Microorganism.*
kijiko kidogo	**teaspoon** *A measure instrument that holds 5 milliliters of fluid.*
kijiko kikubwa	**tablespoon** *An eating utensil that holds 15milliliters of fluid.*
kijimea	**bacteria** *Plural for any organism of the order Eubacteriales.*
kijiwe	**papule** *A small, well-circumscribed elevation of the skin.*
kijiwe katika kibofu cha nyongo	**gallstone** *Calculus produced in the bile duct or gallbladder.*
kijiwe na mkusanyiko wa chokaa mwilini	**calculus** *A stone of minerals that can lead to the blockage of the bile duct or ureters.*
kikohozi	**cough** *Forceful expulsion of air from the lungs.*
kikoma cha uso; kidundu	**forehead** *Section of the face from the hairline to the eyebrows.*
kikombe cha nyonga	**acetabulum** *The cup-shaped cavity with which the head of the femur articulates.*
kikoromeo	**Adam's apple** *A prominence on the anterior neck caused by the thyroid cartilage of the larynx.*
kikuchia; kigozikucha	**hangnail** *A loose piece of skin attached near the medial or lateral nail fold.*
kila	**every** *Each or all possible.*
kila mwaka	**yearly** *Occurring once each year.*
kila siku	**every day** *Each day.*
kila siku nyingine	**every other day** *On alternate days.*
kila wiki	**weekly** *That which occurs every seven days.*

138

Swahili	English
kilango cha arteri kubwa	**aortic valve** *The valve situated between the left ventricle and the aorta.*
kilele	**apex** *The highest point of something.*
kilema	**deformity** *A malformation or imperfection.*
kilengelenge rangi nyekundu	**wheal** *A circumscribed urticarial lesion.*
kimbimbi	**goose bumps** *Cutis anserina.*
kimchango homa	**mite fever** *Synonym of typhus fever.*
kimelea	**parasite** *An organism that lives on or within another organism without benefit to the latter.*
kimeng'enya	**enzyme** *A compound that acts as a catalyst for reactions within cells as assists with digestion outside of cells.*
kimenomeno	**thrush** *Candida albicans*
kimeta	**anthrax** *An infectious disease caused by Bacillus anthracis; there are cutaneous, inhalation and gastrointestinal syndromes.*
kimo cha mtu	**height** *Distance between the bottom of the foot and top of the head.*
kimwili mgawanyo wa kichwa na mwili	**decapitate, to** *The physical separation of the head from the body.*
kina	**deep** *Having significant depth.*
kina cha mshipa donge	**deep vein thrombosis (DVT)** *A blood clot that forms within a vein, typically in the lower extremities.*
kinena	**hypogastrium** *The area of the central abdomen located below the stomach.*
kinena	**inguinal** *Referring to the groin.*
kinena ; manena	**groin** *The genital region.*
kinena misuli kuumia	**groin pull** *A muscle strain in the inguinal region.*
kinena ngiri	**hernia, inguinal** *Protrusion of abdominal-cavity contents through the inguinal canal.*
kingaja	**hand, dorsum** *Back of hand. (kingaja also means bracelet)*
kingalingali	**supine** *Flat on one's back.*
kingamwili	**immune** *Being resistant to an infection.*
kinundu kwenye mfupa	**exostosis** *A bony prominence growing from the surface of a bone.*
kinyaa	**secretion** *The discharge of substances from cells or glands.*
kinyaa cha masikio	**discharge, ear** *Otic secretions.*
kinyaa cha pua	**discharge, nasal** *Nasal secretions.*
kinyaa kupatikana katika kinembe na ngovi; pumba	**smegma** *A thick curdled secretion found around the clitoris and the prepuce.*
kinyaa ya mate	**salivation** *The process of secreting saliva.*
kinyakazi	**wart on clitoris**
kinyesi	**excrement** *Feces.*
kinyesi	**feces** *Excrement.*
kinyesi	**stool** *Feces, excrement.*
kinywa	**mouth** *The orifice on the lower part of the face.*
kioevu nene sana	**sludge** *A viscous fluid.*
kioo	**mirror** *A device used for reflecting an image.*
kipande cha chini cha ncha ya ubongo	**medulla oblongata** *The inferior portion of the brainstem.*

139

Swahili	English
kipande cha katikati kwenye zile ngozi tatu zifunikazo ubongo	**arachnoid** *Refers to that which resembles a spider web.*
kipanulio	**dilator** *An instrument that dilates.*
kipenyo	**perforation** *Presence of a hole.*
kipigo cha mshipa wa damu	**pulse** *The rhythmic throbbing of arteries felt at major vessels.*
kipimadamu	**sphygmomanometer** *Device for measuring blood pressure.*
kipimajoto	**thermometer** *A device used to measure temperature.*
kipimo cha dawa	**dosage** *The amount and frequency a medication is given.*
kipimo kipindi	**dosing interval** *The number of times per unit a medication is given.*
kipindi cha muda baada ya mshtuko wa kifafa	**postictal** *The period of time after a seizure.*
kipindupindu	**cholera** *An infectious disease exhibited by vomiting and diarrhea and caused by Vibrio cholerae.*
kipindupindu ya misuli kwamba ni kutumika kwa karibu jicho	**blepharospasm** *A spasm of the orbicularis oculi muscle that causes closure of the eyelid.*
kipofu	**blind person** *Person with absence of sight.*
kipwepwe	**skin disease that causes red spots**
kiroboto	**flea** *A small wingless insect that feeds on blood of mammals.*
kiseyeye	**scurvy** *A disease of vitamin C deficiency exhibited by bleeding gums.*
kisigino cha mguu	**heel** *Proximal portion of the plantar aspect of the foot.*
kisigino cha mguu-muundi mtihani	**heel-shin test (heel to knee to toe test)** *A test of position sense and coordination; one moves the heel of one foot from the knee on the other foot down to the foot.*
kisimi	**clitoris** *A small erectile body in the anterosuperior aspect of the vulva.*
kisogo; ukosi	**neck, back of (nape)** *Posterior aspect of the neck.*
kisongo	**tourniquet** *A device tied tightly around an extremity to diminish blood flow or blood loss.*
kisonono	**gonorrhea** *A sexually transmitted disease that is exhibited by purulent discharge from the vagina or penis.*
kisonono jicho ugonjwa	**gonorrheal ophthalmia** *An acute purulent conjunctivitis that can occur in neonates within 2-5 days of birth.*
kisugudi	**elbow** *The joint between the humerus and radius/ulna.(right elbow, left elbow)*
kitakapo kaakaa	**cleft palate** *A congenital abnormal opening in the palate.*
kitakapo mdomo	**cleft lip** *A congenital abnormal opening of the lip.*
kitanda mapumziko	**bed rest** *A medical order requiring one to stay in bed.*
kitanda zimefungwa kifaa cha joto	**incubator** *A warming device for infants.*
kitandani	**bedridden** *Term used to indicate one is so ill they cannot get out of bed.*
kitanga cha mkono; kiganja	**hand, palm of**
kitanga cha mkono; kiganja	**palm** *The anterior aspect of the hand.*
kitapo	**shiver** *A trembling.*
kitefute	**cheekbone**

Swahili	English
kitokono; vifupa vitano vya mwisho vya uti wa mgongo vilvyoungamana	**sacrum** *The bone formed by five fused vertebrae that is situated between the two hip bones.*
kitonge	**mass** *Tumor.*
kitovu	**navel** *Umbilicus.*
kitovu	**umbilical cord** *The stalk between the placenta and the unborn infant.*
kitovu	**umbilicus** *The scar that denotes the end of the umbilical cord.*
kitu cha kiasili kwenye mwili kinachopigana na majeraha au na kitu chochoke kigeni mwilini	**histamine** *A chemical responsible for the reaction exhibited when a person has an allergic reaction.*
kitu kama kitambaa chembamba kinachozingira misuli (nyama)	**fascia** *The fibrous sheath enclosing a muscle or organ.*
kitu kama majimaji kilichojaa kwenye macho	**vitreous** *Glass appearance; used to describe the vitreous body of the eye.*
kitu kinachochochea kuongezeka kwa sukari kwenye damu	**glucagon** *A pancreatic enzyme responsible for breakdown of glycogen to glucose.*
kituguta	**maxilla** *The upper jaw that also forms the inferior portion of the orbit and part of the nose.*
kituo cha faya	**health center** *A physical location where patients are treated.*
kiu	**thirst** *The desire to drink.*
kiu isiyoisha	**polydipsia** *Profound thirst.*
kiungo (viungo)	**joint** *Articulation of two adjacent bones.*
kiungo wa bega	**rotator cuff** *The structure around the capsule of the shoulder joint formed by the infraspinatus, supraspinatus, teres minor and subscapularis muscles.*
kiungulia	**dyspepsia** *Indigestion.*
kiungulia	**heartburn** *Synonym of pyrosis.*
kiuno	**lumbar** *Referring to the spinal region inferior to the thoracic spine.*
kiuno maumivu	**coxalgia** *Pain in the hip.*
kiunua	**raise, to** *To lift or bring up.*
kiunzi cha mifupa	**skeleton** *Internal bony framework.*
kivimbe cha mshipa wa damu	**aneurysm** *A condition exhibited by the dilatation of the walls of an artery or vein to form a blood-filled sac.*
kiwaa	**vision, blurred** *Haziness of the visual field.*
kiwaa (kinyenyezi)	**blurred vision** *Low visual acuity. (fuzzy vision)*
kiwambo cha moyo	**diaphragm** *The muscular separation between the thoracic and abdominal cavities.*
kiwambo cha sikio	**ear-drum** *Common term for tympanic membrane.*
kiwambo cha sikio	**tympanic membrane** *The membrane between the external and middle ear.*
kiwango cha moyo zaidi ya 100 mapigo kwa dakika	**tachycardia** *Heart rate higher than physiologic normal.*
kiwasho	**inflammation** *Localized redness, excessive warmth and swelling.*
kiwasho ya pango katika sehemu yo yote mwilini	**sinusitis** *Inflammation of the sinuses.*

141

Swahili	English
kiwasho cha ini	**hepatitis** *Inflammation of the liver.*
kiwasho cha jasho tezi	**hidradenitis** *Inflammation of a sweat gland. When there is purulent discharge it is called hidradenitis suppurativa.*
kiwasho cha matiti	**mastitis** *Inflammation of the breast.*
kiwasho cha mshipa mkubwa	**arteritis** *Inflammation of an artery.*
kiwasho cha shavu	**melitis** *Inflammation of the cheek.*
kiwasho cha uti wa mgongo	**myelitis** *Inflammation of the spinal cord.*
kiwasho na maambukizo of the ufizi	**trench mouth** *Inflammation and ulceration of the gingivae.*
kiwasho ngozi karibu ukucha	**ingrown nail** *Also referred to as onychocryptosis.*
kiwasho wa kidole karibu na ukucha	**paronychia** *Inflammation of the tissue bordering a fingernail*
kiwasho wa kifuko cha machozi	**dacryocystitis** *Inflammation of a lacrimal sac.*
kiwasho wa ubongo na uti wa mgongo	**encephalomyelitis** *Inflammation of the brain and spinal cord.*
kiwasho wa ufizi	**gingivitis** *Inflammation of the gums.*
kiwasho wa ulimi	**glossitis** *Inflammation of the tongue.*
kiwasho ya figo	**nephritis** *A general term meaning inflammation of a kidney that is further categorized depending on the associated pathology.*
kiwasho ya kidaka tonge	**uvulitis** *Inflammation of the uvula.*
kiwasho ya kitovu	**omphalitis** *Inflammation of the umbilicus.*
kiwasho ya koko	**orchitis** *Inflammation of one or both testes.*
kiwasho ya kongosho	**pancreatitis** *Inflammation of the pancreas.*
kiwasho ya koo	**pharyngitis** *Inflammation of the pharynx.*
kiwasho ya macho	**ophthalmia** *Profound inflammation of the eye or its structures.*
kiwasho ya mfuko wa tumbo	**gastritis** *Inflammation of the stomach.*
kiwasho ya misuli	**myositis** *Inflammation of muscle tissue.*
kiwasho ya mrija kutoka figo na kibofu cha mkojo	**ureteritis** *Inflammation of the ureter.*
kiwasho ya mrija kuunganisha ovari ya mji wa mimba	**salpingitis** *Inflammation of the fallopian tubes.*
kiwasho ya mrija wa kutoa mkojo nje kutoka kibofu	**urethritis** *Inflammation of the urethra.*
kiwasho ya neva	**neuritis** *Inflammation of a nerve.*
kiwasho ya ngozi jirani moyo	**pericarditis** *Inflammation of the pericardium.*
kiwasho ya ngozi nyembamba inayofunika sehemu ya nje ya jicho ndani ya kope	**conjunctivitis** *Inflammation of the conjunctiva.*
kiwasho ya ngozi nyembamba inayofunika sehemu ya nje ya jicho ndani ya kope	**pink eye** *Common term for acute contagious conjunctivitis.*
kiwasho ya njia ya haja kubwa	**proctitis** *Inflammation of the rectum.*
kiwasho ya ovari	**oophoritis** *Inflammation of an ovary.*
kiwasho ya sehemu nyeupe ya mboni	**scleritis** *Inflammation of the eyeball.*
kiwasho ya sikio	**otitis** *Inflammation of the ear. (otitis media or otitis externa)*
kiwasho ya ugongo	**encephalitis** *Inflammation of the brain.*

Swahili	English
kiwasho ya ukucha wa kidole cha mkono	**onychia** *Inflammation of the toenail or fingernail matrix.*
kiwasho ya umio	**esophagitis** *Inflammation of the esophagus.*
kiwasho ya umio wa pumzi	**tracheitis** *Inflammation of the trachea.*
kiwasho ya utambi	**peritonitis** *Inflammation of the peritoneum.*
kiwasho ya utumbo mdogo	**enteritis** *Inflammation of the intestines.*
kiwasho ya zoloto	**laryngitis** *Inflammation of the larynx.*
kiwete	**cripple** *A person with a physical disability; not used in polite society.*
kiwewe	**trauma** *A physical injury or emotional shock.*
kiwiko cha mkono; kilimbili	**wrist** *The articulation of the hand and radius/ulna.*
kiwiliwili	**torso** *The trunk of the body.*
kiwinda	**nappy** *Diaper*
kizamani	**obsolete** *No longer in use; antiquated.*
kizinda	**hymen** *A membrane in the vagina.*
kizunguzungu; gumbizi	**dizziness** *Sensation of losing one's balance.*
kizunguzungu; gumbizi	**vertigo** *A sensation of imbalance with many possible causes.*
kizunguzungu; masua	**giddiness** *A tendency to fall or dizziness.*
kodoa macho	**glare** *An angry stare.*
kogo	**occiput** *Back of the head.*
kohozi; belghamu	**sputum** *A mixture of respiratory tract secretions and saliva.*
kojoa damu	**hematuria** *The presence of blood in the urine.*
koko au ovari	**gonad** *A testis or an ovary.*
kokomoka	**retching** *Spasm of the stomach without presence of gastric material.*
koleo	**bistoury; scalpel** *A surgical knife.*
koleo	**scalpel** *A knife used during surgery for incision of skin and tissue.*
koleo	**tongs** *A medical device used for holding or grasping.*
koleo; kitindeo	**forceps** *A surgical instrument, commonly called tweezers.*
kolesteroli	**cholesterol** *A compound or its derivatives are found in cell membranes and precursors to hormones but high levels can cause atherosclerosis.*
kombamwiko	**cockroach** *A beetle-like insect with long legs and antennae.*
kombe	**shellfish** *An aquatic shelled crustacean or mollusk.*
kombeo	**sling** *A device used to give support to an injured extremity.*
kondo kufukuzwa	**expulsion of placenta** *Passage of the placenta out the cervix after childbirth.*
kondo ya nyuma	**afterbirth** *The tissue expelled after the birth of a child that includes the placenta and allied membranes.*
kondo ya nyuma	**placenta** *The vascular tissue that nourishes a fetus through an umbilical cord.*
kondo ya nyuma isiyo mahali pake	**placenta praevia** *A condition in which the placenta covers the cervical os.*
kondomu	**condom** *A covering for the penis or the vagina (female condom) used during sexual intercourse that is meant to reduce the chance of pregnancy or infection.*

Swahili	English
konea	**cornea** *The transparent segment located at the anterior part of the eye.*
kongosho	**pancreas** *A gland that secretes digestive enzymes into the duodenum and insulin and glucagon into the blood.*
koo	**throat** *The anterior aspect of the neck.*
koo; umio	**pharynx** *The membranous cavity from the mouth to esophagus. (umio is sometimes used to describe esophagus at also the larynx)*
kope, ukope	**palpebra, palpebrae** *Eyelid, eyelids.*
kosa	**error** *Mistake or inaccuracy.*
kova tishu	**keloid** *Hypertrophic scar tissue that forms after a minor cut or surgical procedure.*
kovu	**cicatrix (scar)** *New tissue in a healed wound.*
kuahirisha	**postpone, to** *To delay.*
kuambukiza	**contagious** *Description of a disease that can be spread by direct or indirect contact.*
kuambukiza	**infectious** *Contagious.*
kuaminika	**reliable** *Trustworthy.*
kuamka	**awakening** *The state of being conscious.*
kuamua	**ascertain, to** *Synonym of "to determine".*
kuanguka	**collapse** *A physical or mental breakdown.*
kuathiri	**affect** *The expression of emotions or feelings.*
kubwa ateri katika shingo	**carotid** *Referring to the large artery on each side of the neck.*
kubwa au mkubwa	**giant** *Huge or massive.*
kubwa kuliko kawaida	**greater than normal** *Above normal.*
kubwa sana	**enormous** *Very large.*
kubwa ya matumbo	**colon** *The portion of the large intestine that goes from the cecum to the rectum.*
kuchafua	**contaminate, to** *To make impure by exposing to an polluted agent.*
kuchanganyikiwa	**disorientation** *Mental confusion.*
kucheka	**laugh, to**
kuchukua zaidi ya kiasi kinachotakiwa cha dawa	**overdose** *An above normal dose of a medication.*
kuchunguza mauaji	**forensic** *Referring to the scientific method of studying crime.*
kuelekea hatua moja au eneo	**localized** *Toward one point or area.*
kuelekea kichwa	**cephalic** *Towards the head.*
kuendeleza	**sustain, to** *To keep or maintain.*
kuendeleza mafua	**catch a cold** *To come down with a viral upper respiratory tract infection.*
kuenea	**widespread** *Encompassing or spanning.*
kueneza	**saturation** *An amount, expressed in a percentage, that expresses the degree something is absorbed versus the maximal absorption possible.*
kueneza kinyevu na upele unasababishwa na mzio mmenyuko	**urticaria** *A diffuse pruritic macular rash, caused by an allergy.*
kuepukika	**inevitable** *Not preventable.*

144

Swahili	English
kuepukika kuharibika kwa mimba	**abortion, inevitable** *Presence of cervical dilation or ruptured membranes in a pregnancy where the baby is not viable.*
kufa maji	**drown,to** *The process of dying from submerging in and inhaling water.*
kufa; kufariki	**die, to** *To stop living, to expire.*
kufanana mapacha	**identical twins** *Twins from the same zygote.*
kufanyizwa kwa damu	**hemopoiesis** *The production of blood cells from stem cells.*
kufariji maumivu	**relieve, to (pain)** *To make less severe.*
kufikia	**achieve, to** *To complete something one was striving for.*
kufinywa kwa kfua kutokana na jeraha	**traumatic asphyxia** *Cyanotic asphyxia due to trauma. Extravasation of blood into the skin and conjunctivae caused by a sudden increase in venous pressure from a crush injury.*
kufisha	**fatal** *Lethal.*
kufisha saratani ya ngozi	**melanoma** *Malignant cancer, typically found in the skin.*
kufuata	**compliance** *The act of going along with a plan.*
kufukuza shahawa	**ejaculation** *The emission of semen at the moment of sexual climax in a male.*
kufukuzwa	**expulsion** *Evacuation or elimination.*
kufunga	**fasting** *Absence of caloric intake for a specified period.*
kufungwa	**closed**
kufupisha	**shortening** *Notable for having a shorter length.*
kufura kwa kiungo kalichoko nyuma ya kende	**epididymitis** *Inflammation of the duct that moves sperm from the testis to the vas deferens.*
kufura kwa mapafu kutokana na kuwa juu sana	**high altitude pulmonary edema**
kufura kwa matumbo	**gastroenteritis** *A bacterial or viral infection that leads to vomiting and diarrhea.*
kufura kwa nyama nyembamba iunganishayo mifupa na misuli	**tendinitis** *Inflammation of a tendon.*
kufura kwa sikio la ndani	**otitis externa** *Inflammation of the middle ear*
kufura kwa upande wa ndani wa midomo, kinywa na sehemu zinginezo za njia ya pumzi	**angioedema** *Also called angioneurotic edema, it is caused by a histamine reaction. It can produce welts in mild cases but in severe cases can cause swelling of the lips and tongue.*
kufura kwa vena za pumbu	**varicocele** *A cluster of varicose veins in the scrotum.*
kugawanywa katika mashimo madogo	**loculated** *Divided into small cavities.*
kugeuka fudifudi	**pronation** *Turning posteriorly. When the hand is pronated, it is turned medially until the palm is facing posteriorly (when the body was initially in the anatomic position).*
kugeuka nje	**eversion** *To turn outward.*
kuhakikisha	**ensure, to** *To make certain of.*
kuhara mafuta	**steatorrhea** *Excrement with an abnormally high fat content.*
kuhara, kuendesha	**diarrhea, to have** *(verb) The act of having diarrhea.*
kuharibika	**impairment** *A specific disability.*
kuharibika figo kazi	**renal failure** *Diminution of kidney function.*
kuharibika kwa mimba	**miscarriage** *Spontaneous abortion.*
kuhesabu	**count, to** *To determine a number.*
kuhisi kugusa ya mwingine	**sensation** *A perception when one is touched.*

145

Swahili	English
kuhitimu	**qualify** *To become eligible by fulfilling a necessary standard.*
kuhusiana na	**related to** *Causally connected.*
kuibuka	**emergence** *Coming into prominence.*
kuingia kwa ndani	**inversion** *Turning inward.*
kuingiza sindano kupitia kwenye ngozi ya kuvuta maji kutoka ndani ya tumbo	**paracentesis** *A procedure involving aspiration of fluid from the abdominal cavity.*
kuingizwa	**insertion** *The act of inserting something.*
kuingizwa ya kidole ndani ya njia ya haja kubwa wakati wa mitihani ya matibabu	**rectal digital examination** *Use of a gloved finger to assess the rectal vault.*
kuinua	**lift, to** *Raise to a higher level.*
kuizuia	**withhold, to** *To refuse to give something.*
kujadili	**argue, to** *To debate or reason. (quarrel)*
kujiamini	**confidence** *Self-assurance.*
kujifanya kuwa wagonjwa	**malingerer** *A person who feigns illness.*
kujifungua	**parturition** *The process of giving birth.*
kujifunza	**learning** *The intentional acquisition of knowledge.*
kujipenda	**narcissism** *Abnormally excessive self-interest.*
kujisikia	**feel, to** *To perceive or discern.*
kujitolea	**volunteer** *A person who performs work without expecting compensation.*
kujiua makusudi	**suicide** *To kill oneself intentionally.*
kukabiliana	**cope, to** *To deal with a difficult situation.*
kukana	**deny, to** *To reject or repudiate.*
kukasirisha	**provoke, to** *To evoke or elicit.*
kukazana kwa misuli kwenye miguu na mikono	**carpopedal spasm** *A spasm of the carpus and the foot.*
kukinga; kuzuia	**prevent, to** *To stave off or hinder.*
kukohoa damu	**hemoptysis** *Expectoration of blood.*
kukohoa kipindupindu	**coughing fit** *An episode of prolonged, forceful coughing.*
kukojoa	**micturition** *Synonym of urination.*
kukojoa	**voiding** *The act of urinating.*
kukojoa sana	**polyuria** *Abnormal increase in volume of urine excreted.*
kukojoa usiku	**nocturia** *Urination at night.*
kukojosha; dawa inayoongeza mkojo	**diuretic** *Medication which causes an increased excretion of urine.*
kukoma kupumua	**respiratory arrest** *Cessation of breathing.*
kukoma kwa mapafu	**pulmonary embolism** *A sudden blockage of a lung artery frequently emanating from a blood clot in one's leg.*
kukoma kwa moyo kutokana na marilio ya damu hali ya kujazuna	**congestive heart failure** *A diminished cardiac output leading to passive engorgement.*
kukoma kwa uwezo wa moyo kupiga	**cardiac arrest** *Cessation of function of the heart.*
kukoroma (mkoromo)	**snore, to** *To snore or grunt while breathing during sleep. (a snore)*
kukosa au hayupo	**free** *Lacking or absent.*

146

Swahili	English
kukosa homa	**afebrile** *Absence of fever.*
Kukosa mwelekeo	**incoordination** *Absence of smooth, efficient body movement.*
kukosa uwezo wa kudhibiti kukojoa	**incontinence** *Inability to control urination.*
kukosekana hewa	**asphyxia** *A condition exhibited by a lack of oxygen and subsequent loss of consciousness or death.*
kukosekana hewa	**suffocation** *To die from a lack of air or inability to breathe.*
kukosekana kwa	**absence of**
kula	**eat, to** *To consume food.*
kulalana	**sexual intercourse** *The act of copulation.*
kulazimisha pumzi kwa njia ya kufunga mdomo, pua na kidakatonge ili kufanya moyo kupiga polepole	**Valsalva's maneuver** *A technique in which one attempts to exhale with the mouth and nose closed; this equalizes pressure in the ears.*
kulegea	**loose** *Not tight.*
kuleta	**bring, to** *To carry or transport something.*
kuleta kishindo jeraha pamoja	**approximate, to** *To bring together, as in wound margins.*
kuleta kuelekea katikati	**adduction** *To bring toward the midline.*
kulia	**right** *Opposite of left.*
kulia	**sob, to** *To cry uncontrollably.*
kulia	**weep, to** *To shed tears.*
kulia waliyopewa	**right-handed** *Having a preference to use the right hand.*
kulingana na	**according to**
kulisha ndani ya utumbo mdogo	**enteral feeding** *Nutrition supplied via the alimentary canal.*
kulungu kupe	**deer tick** *Ixodes scapularis.*
kumata(mfu)	**dead, to be** *Deceased. (dead person)*
kumba	**heterogenous** *That which originates outside the organism.*
kumbukumbu	**memory** *Ability to remember.*
kumbukumbu	**recollection** *Memory.*
kumbwe cha papasi	**tick bite**
kumeza	**deglutition** *The process of swallowing.*
kumeza	**ingestion** *The intake of food or liquid orally.*
kumeza	**swallow, to** *To cause something to pass down the esophagus.*
kumwaga ngozi	**exfoliation** *The shedding of scales.*
kunguni	**bedbug Cimex lectularius**. *A small insect that is parasitic and hides in clothing or bedding.*
kunja	**flex** *To bend.*
kunung'unika au kulalamika	**querulousness** *Whining or complaining.*
kunusa	**sniff,to** *Short, rapid nasal inhalation. (or to smell)*
kunyimwa	**deprivation** *The lack of a necessity.*
kunyonyesha	**breast feeding** *The process of giving milk to a baby via the nipple.*
kunyoshea	**extend, to** *To expand or stretch out.*
kunywa	**drink, to** *To imbibe.*
kunywa dawa	**take medication, to**
kunywa kiasi kidogo polepole	**sip, to** *To slowly take small drinks of a fluid.*
kuona daktari	**see the doctor, to**

147

Swahili	English
kuondoa	**removal** *The act of removing something.*
kuondoa maiti kutoka kaburini	**exhumation** *To remove a dead body from a grave.*
kuondoa nguo	**disrobe, to** *To remove clothing.*

Swahili-English: kuondoa tishu-moto

Swahili	English
kuondoa tishu zenye madhara	**debridement** *Trimming the dead tissue adjacent to a wound.*
kuondoka hospitali	**hospital discharge** *To leave the hospital.*
kuondolewa kwa bomba kutoka kitundu mwili	**extubation** *The removal of a tube that was in a body orifice.*
kuondolewa kwa maji kutoka tumbo kutumia sindano	**abdominocentesis** *Puncturing of the abdominal wall for drainage purposes.*
kuondolewa kwa maji ya mwili kwa kutumia sindano ya kutathmini kwa ajili ya ugonjwa	**aspiration biopsy** *Removal of fluid from a cavity for pathologic analysis.*
kuondolewa kwa pande la damu	**embolectomy** *The removal of an embolus.*
kuondolewa kwa tishu	**resection** *The removal of tissue.*
kuonekana	**appearance** *The way someone looks or presents.*
kuongeza	**add, to** *To count.*
kuongeza kasi ya	**accelerate** *(To accelerate the healing process).*
kuongeza uzalishaji wa mkojo	**diuresis** *Increased excretion of urine.*
kuongezeka kwa kiwango na kina cha kupumua	**hyperpnea** *Abnormal increase in rate and depth of respiration.*
kuoza kwa jino	**caries** *Referring to decay or death of a tooth.*
kuoza kwa jino	**dental caries** *Decay of teeth.*
kupakana	**proximal** *Situated closer to the center of the body (opposed to that which is farther away, as in distal).*
kupata dawa	**medicine, to get**
kupayuka maneno ovyo	**confabulation** *The fabrication of experiences to compensate for memory loss.*
kupepesa (macho)	**blink, to** *To open and close the eyelid rapidly.*
kupiga cha moyo	**beat** *As in heart beat.*
kupiga teke	**kick, to** *To strike an object with one's foot.*
kupindukia chakula kumeza	**hyperphagia** *Excessive food ingestion.*
kupindukia jasho	**hyperhidrosis** *Excessive perspiration.*
kupinga	**bear, to** *To endure or resist.*
kupinga mitihani kwa sababu ya maumivu	**guarding** *A symptom used to describe a patient resisting an examination because of severe pain; often seen in patients with peritonitis.*
kupingana	**contradictory** *Two elements that are inconsistent.*
kupitia kwa mishipa ya vena	**intravenous** *Within a vein.*
kupitia kwenye ngozi	**transdermal** *Through the skin.*
kupongea	**recover** *(from a serious ailment)*
kupooza cha kaakaa	**palatoplegia** *Paralysis of the palate.*
kupooza kuhusishwa na mitikisiko	**palsy** *Paralysis that is usually associated with tremors.*
kupooza kwa mbili yamefika	**diplegia** *The paralysis of both arms or both legs.*
kupooza kwa muda mfupi	**transient ischemic attack** *Cerebral ischemic changes resulting from transitory hypoperfusion.*

149

Swahili	English
kuporomoka	**drastic** *Having significant effect.*
kupoteza fahamu	**loss of consciousness** *Unresponsive to verbal and tactile stimuli.*
kupoteza hamu ya kula	**anorexia** *The loss of appetite.*
kupoteza kumbukumbu	**amnesia** *The inability to remember past events.*
kupoteza sauti	**aphonia** *The loss of voice.*
kupotoka	**deviation** *Away from the norm.*
kupugawa	**hysteria** *A psychological condition exhibited by uncontrolled emotion or exaggerated manifestations.*
kupumua haraka bila sababu	**hyperventilation** *Rapid and deep respirations.*
kupumua kiwango cha	**respiratory rate** *The number of breaths per minute.*
kupumua kiwango cha juu ya kawaida	**tachypnea** *Breathing faster than normal.*
kupumua kwa shida	**dyspnea** *Difficult breathing.*
kupumua kwa shida wakati kuwekewa chali	**orthopnea** *The inability to breath comfortably except in the upright position.*
kupumuliwa	**expiratory** *Referring to exhalation of air from the lungs.*
kupungua kusikia	**hard of hearing** *Decreased sense of hearing.*
kupungua kwa ukali	**remission** *A decrease in severity or a temporary resolution.*
kupunguza	**alleviate, to**
kupunguza oksijeni ngazi katika damu	**anoxia** *Reduced oxygen levels in body tissues.*
kura ya	**lots of** *An abundance of.*
kuraruka au kukazika kwa misuli au nyama	**sprain** *A joint injury without fracture.*
kurefusha	**lengthening** *Becoming longer.*
kurekebisha	**adjust, to** *To modify a plan.*
kurithi damu machafuko	**hemophilia** *A hereditary bleeding disorder characterized by hemarthroses and deep tissue bleeding as a result of absence of a coagulation factor such as factor VIII.*
kurithiwa	**hereditary** *That which is transmitted genetically*
kurudia	**duplication** *The process of duplicating something.*
kusafisha mfuko wa tumbo	**gastric** *Referring to the stomach.*
kusafisha ndani ya uke na maji au dawa	**douche** *Cleansing of a canal; unless otherwise specified it refers to cleansing of the vaginal canal.*
kusakama kwa hewa mapafuni	**emphysema** *Abnormal enlargement of the airspaces distal to the terminal bronchioles.*
kusema kitembe	**lisping** *A speech problem in which "s" and "z" are pronounced "th".*
kushauri	**advise, to** *To give counsel.*
kushawishi	**induce, to** *Facilitated. When referring to labor, it means medication was given to assist in delivery of the fetus.*
kushoto	**left**
kushuka	**descending** *Moving toward the inferior portion.*
kushusha pumzi	**expiration** *Exhaling.*
kusikia kwa masikio	**hearing** *Auditory perception.*
kusikia misaada	**hearing aid** *A device that fits in the ear used to amplify sound.*

Swahili	English
kusikiliza kwa msaada wa kifaa cha matibabu	**auscultation** *The act of listening to sounds emanating from the body.*
kusinzia	**somnolence** *Drowsiness.*
kusogea	**motor** *Referring to muscles.*
kusokoteka kwa utumbo	**volvulus** *Twisting of the bowel leading to obstruction and sometimes perforation.*
kusujudu	**prostration** *Profound exhaustion.*
kusukutua	**gargle, to** *To rinse one's mouth out and exhale through the liquid.*
kutafuna	**chew, to** *Masticate.*
kutafuna	**mastication** *Chewing.*
kutafuna ya ukucha wa kidole cha mkono	**onychophagia** *Habitually chewing on one's fingernails.*
kutaja	**mention, to** *Refer to or allude to.*
kutanabahi	**conscious** *Being award and being able to respond to one's surroundings.*
kutangua	**cancel, to** *To stop or revoke.*
kutapika	**vomit, to** *To expel gastric contents out the mouth.*
kutapika damu	**hematemesis** *Vomiting blood.*
kutarajia	**expect, to** *To suppose or presume.*
kutatawanya	**scatter** *The degree to which repeated measurements differ.*
kutembea	**ambulation** *Relating to walking.*
kutembea katika hali ile ile kama bata	**waddling gait** *Walking in short steps in a swaying fashion.*
kutenganisha kondo la nyuma na ukuta wa chungu cha mtoto	**placental abruption** *Premature detachment of a normally situated placenta.*
kutengwa eneo	**isolation ward** *A ward where patients with infectious disease are housed.*
kuteseka	**suffer, to** *To be affected by an illness or sickness.*
kutetemeka kwa vifuko vyo moyo	**ventricular fibrillation** *Chaotic and ineffective ventricular contractions.*
kutiba	**cure** *A remedy for a medical illness.*
kutimiza	**accomplish, to** *Achieve.*
kutishia maisha	**life-threatening** *Potentially fatal.*
kutoa mimba	**abortion** (miscarriage) *Premature expulsion of the fetus from the uterus.*
kutojiweza; ulemavu	**disability** *Decreased or impaired mental or physical ability.*
kutoka jasho	**perspiration** *The process of sweating.*
kutokuwa na uwezo wa hoja macho	**ocular paralysis.** *Paralysis of intraocular and extraocular muscles.*
kutokuwa na uwezo wa kuifunga (nywele juu) ya ukope juu ya jicho	**lagophthalmos** *Characterized by the inability to close the eyelid completely over the eye.*
kutokuwa na uwezo wa kutambua sauti kama maneno	**auditory agnosia** *Caused by a temporal lobe lesion, it is characterized by inability to recognize sounds as words.*
kutokuwepo kwa maumivu	**analgesia** *The absence of pain.*
kutokwa na damu ndani ya jicho	**hemophthalmia** *Bleeding within the eye.*

151

Swahili	English
kutokwa na jasho usiku	**night sweats** *Profuse sweating at night occurring with tuberculosis among other conditions.*
kutokwa na makamasi mengi	**coryza** *An acute condition exhibited by copious nasal discharge.*
kutona; kuvuja	**ooze, to** *To slowly leak.*
kutosha	**adequate** *Sufficient.*
kutotulia	**akathisia** *A condition exhibited by motor restlessness and inability to sit quietly.*
kutoweza kukojoa	**urinary retention** *Inadequately emptying the bladder.*
kutoweza kupambanua rangi tofauti	**color blindness** *The inability to distinguish colors.*
kutuliza nafsi	**astringent** *An agent causing contraction of the skin.*
kutunga mimba	**conception** *The act of an egg being fertilized by sperm.*
kuua mwingine	**homicide** *When one person kills another.*
kuumia ; dhara; jeraha	**injury** *A wound, abrasion or contusion.*
kuumia kwa ubongo	**head trauma** *Any injury to the brain.*
kuumika	**blood-letting** *The removal of blood from a patient with the thought it would cure or prevent disease.*
kuumwa na jino	**toothache** *Dental pain.*
kuundwa kwa kifuko ya upasuaji	**marsupialization** *Creation of a surgical pouch.*
kuvimba katika mwisho wa uume	**balanitis** *Inflammation of the glans of the penis.*
kuvimba kwa mefereji na vyombo vya maji ya mwilini	**lymphangitis** *Inflammation of the lymph vessels.*
kuvimba kwa sehemu nyororo, laini iliyoko katikati ya jino	**pulpitis** *Dental pulp inflammation.*
kuvimba kwa tezi kwa wanaume	**prostatitis** *Inflammation of the prostate gland.*
kuvimba matumbo kubwa	**colitis** *Inflammation of the colon.*
kuvimba nyongo	**cholecystitis** *Inflammation of the gallbladder.*
kuvimba tezi	**adenitis** *The inflammation of a gland.*
kuvimba tumbo	**swollen (distended) abdomen**
kuvimba utando wa kamasi; mafua	**catarrh** *Inflammation of a mucous membrane.*
kuvimba wa ngozi	**dermatitis** *Non-specific inflammation of the skin.*
kuvuja	**leakage** *Unintentional escape of gas or fluid.*
kuvuja kwa damu	**hemorrhage** *Bleeding from a damaged blood vessel.*
kuvunjika	**break** *A common term for a fracture in a bone.*
kuvunjika	**rupture** *An instance of bursting suddenly.*
kuvunjika ambako hakupenyi mfupa kabisa	**fracture, greenstick** *A spiral fracture.*
kuvunjika kwa chakula katika matumbo	**digestion** *The process of enzymatic breakdown of food in the alimentary canal.*
kuvunjika kwa rangi nyekundu ya damu	**hemolysis** *Breakdown of hemoglobin.*
kuvunjwa mkono	**broken (arm)** *Fracture of the arm.*
kuvuta	**pull, to** *To exert force on something.*
kuvuta (sigara)	**smoke, to** *To inhale on a cigarette.*

152

Swahili	English
kuvuta pumzi	**inhalation** *The act of breathing in.*
kuvuta pumzi	**inspiration** *Drawing in a breath.*
kuvuta ya mfupa kutibu mfupa uliovunjika (kutumia mfumo wa kapi)	**skeletal traction** *Use of a pulley system to reduce a fracture.*
kuwa imefungwa	**obstructed** *To be blocked or halted.*
kuwa kitapo	**shake, to** *To tremble uncontrollably.*
kuwa mipaka ya kudumu	**demarcation** *Having a fixed boundary.*
kuwa na kiasi kidogo cha hewa ya oxygen	**hypoxia** *Diminished oxygen content.*
kuwa na kujiwe figo	**nephrolithiasis** *A calculus in the kidney.*
kuwa wa wasiwasi	**anxious** *Experiencing nervousness or unease.*
kuwadhuru	**injure, to** *To hurt or to wound.*
kuwafahamisha	**acquaint, to** *To make someone familiar with something.*
kuwasiliana na	**contact** *The touching of two bodies or a person who has been exposed to a contagious disease.*
kuwekewa gorofa katika kitanda	**decubitus** *Laying flat in bed or dorsal decubitus. (lateral decubitus is flat and on one's side)*
kuyapatia	**endow, to** *To supply or provide for.*
kuzaa	**bear, to** *To give birth to a child.*
kuzaa (kujifungua kusaidiwa kwa koleo)	**delivery** *The process of giving birth. (forceps delivery)*
kuzaa chini	**bearing down** *As in during labor.*
kuzalima alama	**nevus** *A benign, well-circumscribed growth of tissue of congenital origin.*
kuzaliwa abnormality: kupita kiasi kavu ngozi	**ichthyosis** *A congenital anomaly exhibited by excessively dry, thick skin.*
kuzaliwa makosa	**birth defect** *A congenital anomaly.*
kuzibwa kwa mfereji wa damu na kidonge cha damu iliyoshikana	**embolus** *A blood clot, air bubble or fatty deposit that cause obstruction of a vessel.*
kuzingatia	**comply, to** *Adhere to.*
kuzira au epuka	**abstain, to** *To give up or to stop.*
kuzirai	**blackout** *Common term for loss of consciousness.*
kuzorota	**deterioration** *Worsening in one's medical condition.*
kuzuiwa kwa damu kufikia sehemu fulani za ubongo	**cerebrovascular accident (stroke)** *A decrease in level of consciousness and paralysis caused by a cerebrovascular thrombosis, hemorrhage or vasospasm.*
kuzungumza ambayo nai vigumu kuelewa lakini kueleweka	**slurring** *Indistinct yet comprehensible speech.*
kwa kinywa (kwa kunena)	**orally** *By mouth. (verbally)*
kwa sababu ya	**owing to** *On account of.*
kwanza kidonda ya kaswende	**chancre** *The initial ulcer that is seen with primary syphilis.*
kwanza waliozaliwa kinyesi kuchanganywa na maji yanayozunguka kijusi	**meconium** *The first newborn feces which are green.*
kwanza ya hedhi kipindi	**menarche** *The time of the initial menstrual period.*

153

Swahili	English
kwanza ya sehemu ya utumbo mdogo	**duodenum** *The portion of the small bowel between the stomach and jejunum.*
kwapa	**armpit** *A common term for axilla.*
kwapa	**axilla** *The hollow beneath the arm.*
kweli	**indeed** *As a matter of fact.*
kwenda hospitali	**go to the hospital, to**
kwenda kwa daktari	**go to the doctor, to**
kwikwi; chechevu	**hiccup** *Involuntary spasm of the diaphragm with sudden closure of the glottis; this causes a characteristic cough.*
kwingo cha moyo	**heart rate** *Number or cardiac contractions per minute.*
ladha	**taste** *Sensation of flavor perceived in one's mouth.*
laini	**soft** *Easy to mold or compress.*
lainisha kwa mafuta	**lubricant** *Emollient.*
lazima	**mandatory** *Obligatory.*
lengelenge	**blister** *Common term for bulla.*
lengelenge	**vesicle** *A blister.*
lengo	**target** *An objective towards which efforts are directed.*
lenzi	**lens** *The transparent chamber between the posterior chamber and the vitreous body.*
licha ya	**despite** *Notwithstanding.*
limfosaiti	**lymphocyte** *A white blood cell produced by the lymph tissue.*
limfu	**lymph** *A transparent and sometimes opalescent fluid that flows in the lymph channels.*
limfu nodi	**lymph node** *An area of organized lymphatic tissue.*
limfu, aina nyingi	**lymphoma** *A malignant disease of the lymph system, Hodgkin's lymphoma for example.*
lisilo	**irrelevant** *Not pertinent.*
losinofili	**eosinophil** *A cell with eosin stain used to designate a type of leukocyte that is elevated during allergic reactions.*
maabara ya matokeo	**lab result** *The data obtained from a laboratory test.*
maalum	**specific** *Clearly defined.*
maambukizi na kiwasho ya mfupa	**osteomyelitis** *Inflammation of the bone or bone marrow because of a microorganism.*
Maambukizi Rickettsiae ulioonyeshwa na upele, homa na kuumwa na misuli, na maumivu ya kichwa	**typhus fever** *A rickettsiae infection exhibited by rash, fever, headache and myalgia.*
maambukizi ya konea unasababishwa na Klamidia	**trachoma** *An infection of the cornea and conjunctiva caused by Chlamydia.*
maambukizi ya kuwashirikisha ovari na mfuko wa uzazi	**pelvic inflammatory disease** *Generally a bacterial infection affecting a woman with potential involvement of the uterus, fallopian tubes, ovaries and cervix.*
maambukizi ya vimelea ya sikio	**otomycosis** *Fungal infection of the ear.*
maana	**meaningless** *Having no significance.*
maandishi	**compendium** *A concise summary about a subject.*
mabadiliko	**alteration** *The process of change or modification.*
mabaya	**detrimental** *Harmful.*
machafu	**hazy** *Cloudy.*

154

Swahili	English
machafuko	**confusion** *Disorientation.*
machela	**stretcher** *A device used to carry a patient in the supine position.*
machozi	**lacrimal fluid** *Fluid secreted by the lacrimal gland.*
machozi	**tear**s Fluid expelled from the eyes during crying.
madawa ambayo husababisha usingizi	**hypnotic** *Sleep inducing agent.*
madhii; shahawa	**semen**
madini	**iodine** *A chemical used as an antiseptic and a deficiency of it can lead to goiter.*
madoa meupe juu ngozi	**vitiligo** *The appearance of non-pigmented white patches on otherwise normal skin; hair is usually white in the affected areas.*
maendeleo	**progressive** *Developing gradually.*
maendeleo ya kupoteza uzito	**marasmus** *Progressive weight loss and emaciation.*
mafuta	**fat** *A greasy or oiling substance naturally occurring in the body.*
mafuta donge	**lipoma** *A benign tumor consisting of fat cells.*
magodoro	**mattress** *A fabric case filled with material, used for sleeping.*
magonjwa Parkinson	**Parkinson's disease** *A progressive neuromuscular disease exhibited by masklike facial expression, resting tremor, cogwheel rigidity and abnormal gait.*
magonjwa ya kuambukiza na sifa ya unyonge na utvidgningen ya limfu nodi	**mononucleosis** *An infectious disease exhibited by malaise and lymphadenopathy.*
magonjwa ya mlipuko	**epidemiology** *The study of the incidence, development and control of disease.*
mahadhi	**rhythm** *The pattern or cadence.*
mahali	**site** *Location.*
mahoka	**mania** *A mental disorder exhibited by hyperexcitability, delusions and euphoria.*
maisha	**lifetime** *Duration of a person's life.*
maisha marefu	**longevity** *Long life.*
maiti	**cadaver** *A dead body.*
majeruhi	**casualty** *A person who is killed or seriously injured.*
maji	**water** *A colorless, odorless liquid.*
maji katika sehemu ya mbele ya jicho	**aqueous humor** *The fluid between the cornea and lens, anterior to the globe.*
maji mkusanyiko ndani ya mapafu	**pulmonary edema** *Characterized by abnormal fluid buildup in the lungs.*
maji uti wa mgongo	**CSF** *Abbreviation for cerebrospinal fluid.*
maji ya kunywa	**drinking water** *Water clean enough to ingest orally.*
maji ya ulaji	**fluid intake** *The amount of oral consumption plus the amount of intravenous fluids administered.*
maji yanayozunguka kijusi; ugiligili ya amnioni (kuzunguka kijusi wakati wa mimba)	**amniotic fluid** *The fluid surrounding the fetus.*
maji yenye chumvi	**saline** *A solution of sodium chloride.*
majibu	**reaction** *A response to an action.*
majibu ya chumvi na dutu	**anaphylaxis** *An exaggerated response to a foreign substance.*

Swahili	English
makazi yao	**displacement** *Movement from normal position.*
makelele au sauti za mifupa iliyovunjika hasa wakati inapokwaruzana (2)	**crepitus** *A noise heard when one auscultates the lungs that is similar to the sound of rubbing hair between one's fingers.(1) It is also considered the sound of two broken bones rubbing together. (2)*
makende yanapojipinda ndani ya ule mfuko wake	**testicular torsion** *Rotation of the spermatic cord resulting in testicular ischemia.*
makisio ya maendeleo ya ugonjwa	**prognosis** *The likely course of a disease.*
makohoo	**expectoration** *The presence of sputum that has been coughed out.*
makubaliano	**agreement** *Accordance in opinion or feeling.*
makubwa huzuni	**melancholia** *Profound sadness.*
makubwa ya ugonjwa wa akili	**psychosis** *A profound mental disorder that can include delusions and hallucinations.*
malalaliko	**complaint** *Grievance.*
malale	**sleeping sickness** *Also called Trypanosomiasis, this disease is caused by a parasitic protozoa and transmitted by the tsetse fly.*
malale	**trypanosomiasis** *A disease caused by a protozoa of the genus Trypanosoma that can cause sleeping sickness and Chagas' disease.*
malaria (mkojo ni rangi nyekundu-nyeusi)	**blackwater fever** *A term used to describe the fever associated with malaria when the urine is reddish-black.*
malaya	**prostitute** *A person who exchanges goods or services for sex.*
malendalenda	**stool, watery with mucous**
malengelenge sehemu za siri	**genital herpes** *A sexually transmitted infection caused by herpes simplex.*
malengelenge; manawa	**herpes** *A skin condition exhibited by formation of clustered vesicular lesions; herpes simplex is at times referred to, albeit incompletely, as herpes.*
manii	**sperm** *Short term for spermatozoon.*
maombi	**application** *The forms one fills out to obtain a grant.*
maombi ya banzi	**brace, to** *Application of a splint.*
maombolezo	**mourning** *A period of grieving.*
maoni	**comment** *A remark providing an opinion.*
maono	**vision** *State of being able to see.*
mapafu	**edema** *Extravascular fluid accumulation.*
mapema	**premature** *Occurring earlier than expected.*
mapotofu	**aberrant** *Different than normal.*
mapumziko	**rest** *Relaxation or respite.*
mara mbili	**two times** *One action being done on two occasions.*
mara mbili	**double** *Twice the size, quantity or strength.*
mara mbili maono katika jicho mmoja tu	**monodiplopia** *Double vision in only one eye.*
mara mbili ya maono	**diplopia** *Double vision.*
maradhi	**morbidity** *The state of disease.*
maradhi ya mti	**gangrene** *Tissue death from either impaired blood flow or an infection.*
maradhi; ugonjwa	**disease** *Malady or disorder.*

Swahili	English
marekebisho	**adjustment** *A modification of a plan.*
masikio, pua na koo	**ENT** *Abbreviation for ears, nose and throat.*
matako (tako); makalio	**buttocks (buttock)** *The bilateral region covering the gluteal muscles.*
matapisha	**emesis** *Vomit (noun)*
matapishi	**vomit** *The gastric contents that are expelled through the mouth.*
mate	**saliva** *The watery liquid secreted by the salivary glands.*
mate	**spit** *A term used to describe saliva that is ejected from the mouth.*
matege	**bow-legged person**
matende	**elephantiasis** *A condition caused by nematode parasites leading to lymphatic obstruction and limb or scrotal swelling.*
matibabu chombo kutumika kukagua uke	**speculum** *A device used to open a canal for inspection. (vaginal speculum)*
matibabu tathmini	**assessment** *An medical evaluation.*
matone kwa dakika	**drops per minute** *Refers to iv fluid rate.*
matumbo	**intestine** *A general term used for the section of bowel from the stomach to the anus.*
matumbo kizuizi	**intestinal obstruction** *Blockage of the intestine by mass or volvulus.*
matumizi ya dawa ya kufanya mtu usingizi wakati wa upasuaji	**anesthetic** *A chemical that produces anesthesia.*
matumizi ya kawaida ya kuapika	**cyclical vomiting** *Periods of recurrent vomiting with no apparent pathologic cause and the person has a normal state of health between the episodes.*
matumizi ya kawaida ya maambukizi ya bakteria na homa	**relapsing fever** *A recurrent bacterial infection, with fever, caused by Spirochetes.*
matumizi ya sindano ya kuondoa maji kutoka tumboni	**amniocentesis** *Transabdominal aspiration of amniotic fluid.*
maudhui	**content** *What something is made up of.*
maumivu	**pain** *Physical suffering or discomfort.*
maumivu au ugonjwa unaoletwa na minni vinavyoenezwa na kupe	**tularemia** *An infectious disease caused by Francisella tularensis. The symptoms range from mild constitutional complaints to septic shock.*
maumivu cha enda choo	**dyschezia** *Pain experienced during defecation.*
maumivu cha kichwa	**headache** *Cephalgia.*
maumivu cha kichwa upande mmoja; kipandauso	**migraine** *An episodic, unilateral headache accompanied by nausea.*
maumivu cha matiti	**mastodynia** *Breast pain.*
maumivu katika mguu kwamba imekuwa ulikatwa	**phantom limb pain** *Pain sensed in an area where one has had an amputation as though the limb is still present.*
maumivu makai; uchungu	**agony** *Anguish or torment.*
maumivu makali pamoja neva	**neurapraxia** *Paralysis from nerve injury but no degeneration of the nerve.*
maumivu wa ulimi	**glossodynia** *Tongue pain.*
maumivu ya hedhi	**dysmenorrhea** *Pain during menstruation.*
maumivu ya koko	**orchialgia** *Testicular pain.*
maumivu ya koo	**sore throat** *Common term for pharyngitis.*

157

Swahili	English
maumivu ya kuhusishwa na kumeza	**odynophagia** *Pain associated with swallowing.*
maumivu ya meno	**odontalgia** *Tooth pain.*
maumivu ya mgongo	**back pain** *Discomfort on the dorsal surface of the torso.*
maumivu ya misuli	**myalgia** *Muscle pain.*
maumivu ya neva	**neuropathy** *Structural of pathologic changes of the peripheral nervous system.*
maumivu ya sikio	**earache** *Pain associated with the ear.*
maumivu ya sikio	**otalgia** *Ear pain.*
mauti	**death** *The action of dying.*
mauti	**lethal** *Deadly.*
mauti dosi	**lethal dose** *The amount of a drug required to cause death.*
mavu	**wasp** *Any one of a winged hymenopterous insects.*
maziwa ya ng'ombe	**cow's milk**
mba	**dandruff** *Dead skin found in the hair.*
mbali	**apart** *Separated by a distance.*
mbali na	**away from** *Separated from.*
mbali; mbail na katikati	**distal** *Situated away from the center of the body.*
mbavu	**ribs** *A series of curved paired boney articulations protecting the thorax. (In Swahili, ubavu is also used for "side", "hip" & rib.)*
mbaya pumzi	**halitosis** *Foul odor emanating from the mouth.*
mbaya ya athari	**adverse effect** *In reference to medication use, it is an undesirable consequence of the drug.*
mbaya ya athari kutokana na kutumia dawa	**drug reaction** *Typically refers to an adverse effect of medication.*
mbaya ya tatizo lililopo	**exacerbation** *Worsening of an existing problem.*
mbaya zaidi	**worsen, to** *To deteriorate.*
mbele	**anterior** *Toward the front.*
mbele	**forwards** *Towards the front.*
mbele	**ventral** *Referring to the underside but in humans, a ventral hernia, for example, refers to an abdominal hernia.*
mbele ya protini katika mkojo	**proteinuria** *The presence of protein in the urine.*
mbele ya sikio	**preauricular** *Anterior to the ear.*
mbenuko	**bulge** *A protuberance on a flat surface.*
mbenuko	**tuberosity** *A protuberance. For instance the iliac tuberosity is a prominence on the surface of the ilium.*
mbenuko wa jicho	**exophthalmos** *Protrusion of one or both eyeballs.*
mbenuko wa jicho	**proptosis oculi** *Synonym of exophthalmos; bulging of the eye.*
mbenuko ya mfuko wa uzazi kwa njia ya uke	**prolapse of the uterus** *Eversion of the uterus through the vagina.*
mbu yanayotokana na ugonjwa wa homa na maumivu	**dengue** *A mosquito-borne viral disease exhibited by fever and joint pain.*
mbulanga	**hyperpigmentation, skin disease causing** *General term to describe skin darkening.*
mbweu	**belch** *Eructation.*
mbweu	**eructation** *Belch or burp.*
mchafu kunusa jasho	**bromidrosis** *Foul smelling perspiration.*

158

Swahili	English
mchana	**noon** *The 12 o'clock mid-day hour.*
mchanga	**baby** *A newborn.*
mchanganyaji dawa	**pharmacist** *A professional who prepares and sells medicine through various systems, including governmental organizations like the Veterans Administration.*
mchango; mnyoo	**worm** *Any of long, slender, legless, soft-bodied invertebrates.*
mchochota	**pruritus** *A general term for conditions exhibited by itching.*
mchochota wa kibofu cha mkojo	**cystitis** *Inflammation of the urinary bladder.*
mchochota wa kope; kikope	**blepharitis** *Inflammation of the eyelids.*
mchomo cha tumbo	**pyrosis** *Synonym for heartburn.*
mdomo	**labium** *Referring to any lip shaped structure.*
mdomo	**oral** *Relating to the mouth.*
mdomo uzazi wa mpango	**oral contraceptive** *Tablet taken by mouth to prevent pregnancy.*
mduara	**circumference** *The distance around an object or part.*
mdudu	**bug** *Insect.*
meno	**dental** *Referring to teeth.*
meno bandia	**denture** *A frame that holds artificial teeth.*
meno msongano	**impaction, tooth** *A tooth that does not erupt because adjacent teeth prevent it.*
mfadhaiko; usononi	**depression** *A medical condition exhibited by profound despondency.*
mfereji unaounganisha sikio na koo	**eustachian tube** *The muscular canal that connects the tympanic membrane with the pharynx*
mfereji wenye umbo la	**cochlea** *The essential organ of hearing which is in a spiral form.*
mfinyo	**constriction** *Circumferential tightening*
mfuko wa pumbu; korodani	**scrotum** *The sac which contains the testes.*
mfuko wa ya mimba	**amnion** *The membrane lining the placenta which produces the amniotic fluid.*
mfupa	**bone** *Skeletal tissue formed by osteoblasts.*
mfupa mkubwa katika sehemu ya chini ya mguu	**tibia** *The larger of two long bones in the lower leg.*
mfupa laini kwenye kiungo cha goti ambao una sura ya nusu mwezi	**meniscus** *A thin cartilage between joint surfaces.*
mfupa ndogo katika mguu chini	**fibula** *The smaller of two bones in the lower leg.*
mfupa wa kidari	**sternum** *Commonly called the breast bone, it consists of the corpus, manubrium and xiphoid process.*
mfupa wa kifundo cha mguu	**talus** *The most superior tarsal bone that articulates with the tibia.*
mfupa wa kinena	**pubis** *The anterior inferior part of the hip bone on each side that articulates at the pubic symphysis.*
mfupa wa kisigino	**calcaneus** *Commonly called the heel bone.*
mfupa wa kitako	**ischium** *The inferoposterior portion of the pelvis.*
mfupa wa mkono katikati ya kiko na bega	**humerus** *The long bone in the upper arm.*
mfupa wa paja	**femur** *The long bone in the thigh.*

159

Swahili	English
mfupa yanayozunguka jicho	**orbit** *The bony structure enclosing the eyeball.*
mfupi upana fuvu	**bradycardia** *Lower than normal cardiac rate measured in beats per minute.*
mgogoro	**crisis** *A turning point in the treatment of a disease.*
mgongo	**spine** *The spinal column or a thorny protrusion.*
mgonjwa	**patient** *The client being treated for a medical or surgical condition.*
mguu	**leg** *One of two lower extremities.*
mguu wa mapafu	**lower extremity edema** *Interstitial edema of the legs.*
mibinu for kuzuia mimba ndani ya mfuko la uzazi	**intrauterine contraceptive device (IUD)** *A device used to physically prevent the implantation of a fertilized ovum.*
mifupa midogo ya mguu	**cuneiform** *The three bones between the navicular bone and the metatarsals.*
mifupa ya vidole vya mikono ama vya miguu	**phalanges** *The long bones of the fingers or toes.*
migogoro	**conflict** *Dispute or disagreement.*
mijadala kamba	**vocal cords** *Paired folds of mucous membranes stretched across the larynx.*
mimba	**fetus** *Medical term for the infant prior to birth.*
mimba iliyo nje ya mji wake	**ectopic pregnancy** *A pregnancy that is not intrauterine.*
mimba zaidi ya mara moja	**multigravida** *A woman who has been pregnant more than once.*
minya	**squeeze, to** *To apply pressure.*
mishipa midogu ya damu ambapo mabadilishano ya hewa kati ya damu na viungo vya mwili hutokeo	**capillary** *A vessel that connects arterioles to venules.*
mishtuko	**convulsions** *An involuntary series of tonic and clonic movements.*
misingi	**underlying** *Causative, unexposed, or fundamental.*
misogeo ya kwanza ya mtoto tumboni	**quickening** *Signs of life noted by a mother as the fetus moves.*
misuli	**muscle** *A band if fibrous tissue that can contract.*
misuli kati ya mbavu	**muscle, intercostal**
misuli mishazari	**muscle, oblique**
misuli nyama ya moyo	**myocardium** *The middle layer of the heart wall.*
misuli nyama za matako	**gluteal or gluteus muscle** *A paired set of three muscles, the gluteus maximus, medius and minimus, that all have origins in the ilium and insertions in the femur. (buttocks)*
misuli nyama za mguu upande wa nyuma	**hamstrings** *Tendons of the posterior thigh.*
misuli wa paja	**muscle, quadriceps**
misuli wa ukosi	**muscle, trapezius**
misuli ya bega	**muscle, deltoid**
misuli ya fumbatio	**muscle, abdominal**
misuli ya kifua	**muscle, pectoral**
misuli ya matako	**muscle, gluteus maximus**
misuli ya mgongo wa juu	**muscle, latissimus dorsi**
misuli ya paja	**quadriceps** *The anterior thigh muscle composed of four muscles.*

160

Swahili	English
misuli:nyama za upande wa nyuma wa miguu	**gastrocnemius** *A large muscle in the lower leg, responsible for ankle plantar flexion, that is attached to the distal femur and achilles tendon.*
mito	**pillow** *An encased fabric covering soft material used for a cushion.*
miwani	**eyeglasses** *Eye wear used for cosmetic or prescription purposes.*
mizani	**scale** *A device to check a person's weight.*
mjamzito	**pregnant woman**
mji wa mimba	**uterus** *The hollow organ in the female pelvis where a fertilized ovum embeds and grows.*
mkali	**bright** *Giving out a lot of light.*
mkali	**sharp (pain)** *When describing pain, a piercing sensation.*
mkamba	**bronchitis** *Inflammation of the mucous membranes of the bronchioles that causes bronchospasm and cough.*
mkanda wa jeshi	**herpes zoster; shingles** *A unilateral vesicular rash along one dermatome and caused by inflammation of a posterior nerve root by "the chicken pox virus".*
mkanda wa jeshi	**shingles** *A reactivation of herpes zoster.*
mkasi	**scissors** *A cutting instrument with two blades, joined at the middle.*
mkazo	**stress** *Strain or pressure.*
mkia	**caudal** *Referring to a cauda.*
mkojo	**urine** *The fluid concentrated by the kidneys and expelled via the urethra.*
mkojo sababu ya udhaifu	**urinary incontinence** *Involuntary micturition.*
mkondo au mtiririko	**current** *Flow or stream.*
mkongojo	**crutch** *Long metal or wooden stick used for support while walking.*
mkono	**arm** *One of two upper extremities.*
mkono	**hand** *The upper extremity distal to the wrist.*
mkono au mguu	**extremity** *Refers to one arm or one leg.*
mkono au mguu	**member** *Referring to an extremity (arm or leg).*
mkono wa kulia	**hand, right**
mkono wa kushoto	**hand, left**
mkundu	**anal** *Near or referring to the anus.*
mkundu	**anus** *The body opening distal to the rectum.*
mkunga	**midwife** *A person trained to assist in childbirth.*
mkunjo ya ngozi	**skin fold** *An overlapping of skin formed by subcutaneous tissue.*
mkusanyiko wa maji katika ubongo	**hydrocephalus** *The excessive accumulation of cerebral spinal fluid in the brain causing enlargement of the head.*
mkuwadi	**impotence** *Inability to act or inability to achieve a penile erection.*
mkwaruzo	**abrasion** *Superficial skin injury.*
mkwaruzo	**scratch** *A long, narrow superficial wound.*
mlezi	**caregiver** *A person who provides care to another.*
mlipuko	**epidemic** *Ubiquitous development of an infectious disease.*
mluzi	**whistle, to** *To make a high pitch noise by forcing air through the lips.*

Swahili	English
mmomonyoko wa tishu	**erosion** *The gradual destruction of surface tissue.*
mnong'ono	**whisper** *Speech in a volume that is barely discernible.*
mnururisho	**radiation** *1. The emission of energy in the form of electromagnetic waves. 2. Divergence from a common point.*
mochari	**morgue** *A room where deceased patients are housed until sent to a funeral home.*
moja moja maumivu makali ya kichwa	**cluster headache** *A unilateral, severe, recurrent headache.*
moja moja usoni kupooza (neva ya fuvu tatizo)	**Bell's palsy** *Unilateral facial paralysis related to dysfunction of the seventh cranial nerve.*
moja tu ya	**single** *Only one.*
mojawapo ya zile njia mbili kubwa za hewa kutoka kwenye pipa la hewa	**bronchus** *The major air channels that bifurcate from the distal trachea.*
monosaiti	**monocyte** *A leukocyte with an oval nucleus and grey cytoplasm.*
moto	**hot** *Very warm.*

162

Swahili-English: moyo-ugonjwa wa Crohn

Swahili	English
moyo	**cardiac** *Referring to the heart.*
moyo	**heart** *Muscular organ that pumps blood thru the circulatory system.*
moyo msinung'unike	**heart murmur** *An abnormal heart sound usually related to valvular disease.*
moyo-mapafu kufufuliwa	**cardiopulmonary resuscitation** *Use of artificial means to support respiration and circulation.*
mpango	**scheme** *A program or plan.*
mpindanowa misuli	**cramp** *A painful contraction of muscles.*
mrija kutoka figo na kibofu cha mkojo	**ureter** *The conduit between each kidney and the urinary bladder.*
mrija kuunganisha ovari ya mji wa mimba	**fallopian tubes** *Either of a pair of long narrow ducts located in a female's abdominal cavity that transport the male sperm cells to the egg.*
mrija kuunganisha ovari ya mji wa mimba	**oviduct** *The channel which an ovum passes from the ovary.*
mrija wa kusafisha tumbo kuingizwa kupitia pua	**nasogastric tube** *A tube that is inserted into the nose with the distal tip in the stomach; it is used for irrigation or drainage of gastric contents.*
mrija wa kutoa mkojo nje kutoka kibofu	**urethra** *The canal connecting the urinary bladder with the outside of the body.*
mrija wa nyongo	**bile ducts** *The structures that are conduits for passage of bile from the liver and gallbladder to the duodenum.*
mruba	**leech** *An annelid used in some tropical regions for drawing out blood; they have an anticoagulant effect locally and have been attached to digits of persons with acute peripheral ischemia.*
msamba	**perineum** *The area between the anus and scrotum or anus and vulva.*
msawazisho	**equilibrium** *When opposing forces are in balance.*
mshikamano	**affinity** *To have a natural liking for.*
mshipa inakuwa miembamba	**vasoconstriction** *The process of making the blood vessels smaller which increases blood pressure.*
mshipa inapanuka	**vasodilatation** *The process of making the blood vessels larger which decreases blood pressure.*
mshipa mkubwa	**artery** *Vessel that carries oxygenated blood from the heart to the periphery.*
mshipa mkubwa wa damu wa upande wa kushoto wa moyo	**aorta** *The large artery originating at the left ventricle and going to the pelvis where it bifurcates.*
mshipa unaopeleka damu kwenye misuli ya moyo	**coronary vessel** *Referring to a coronary artery.*
mshipa wa damu	**blood stream** *Common term or the arterial or venous systems.*
mshipa wa fahamu	**nerve** *A fibrous band made up of axons and dendrites that connects the nervous systems with other organs.*
mshipa wa kisigino	**Achilles tendon** *Also called calcaneal tendon; tendon with insertion at the gasrocnemius & soleus into the tuberosity of the calcaneus*

163

Swahili	English
mshono kutumika kufunga chombo damu	**ligature** *A thread used to tie a vessel.*
mshono wa kuziba jeraha	**suture** *Thread used for sewing together a wound.*
mshtuko	**strain** *As in a muscle strain.*
mshtuko wa moyo	**myocardial infarction** *The death of myocardial tissue as a result of an interruption in flow to the region supplied by a coronary vessel.*
mshtuko; kuathiriwa kwa uhusiano/ushirikiano wa kawaida wa kiungo	**dislocation** *The displacement of a bone when referring to an articulation. (sprain, dislocate, startle)*
mshumaa	**candle** *A cylindrical piece of wax with a central wick.*
msiba	**bereavement** *The sorrow one feels with the loss of a loved one.*
msimamo au hali	**standing** *Position or status.*
msokoto wa tumbo	**colic** *Acute abdominal pain.*
msongano kwa kinyesi	**fecal impaction** *The presence of hard excrement in the rectum that requires manual removal.*
msuguano	**friction** *Grating or rasping.*
msukumo wa damu; shinikizo la damu	**blood pressure** *Written as the measurement in mmHg at the time of systole of the left ventricle over the time of diastole.*
msumeno	**saw** *A hand or power-driven tool used for cutting.*
mtaalamu katika matatizo ya lugha na akizungumza	**speech therapist** *A person trained to assist people with speech and language disorders.*
mtai	**cut** *An incision.*
mtazamaji	**monitor** *A person that observes a process or a monitoring device.*
mtazamo	**gaze** *Steady, intent look.*
mtazamo	**glance** *A brief look at something.*
mti; mlezi	**scrofula** *Cervical tuberculous lymphadenitis. (Mlezi also means guardian in Swahili)*
mtikiso	**concussion** *Head trauma resulting in temporary loss of consciousness.*
mtiririko	**flow** *Movement in a continuous stream.*
mto	**cushion** *A pillow or stuffed pad used to sit on.*
mtoki dalili ya kaswende elimu ya juu	**gumma** *A soft granulomatous tumor of the skin or cardiovascular system seen in tertiary syphilis.*
mtoto (kiume, kike)	**child** *A person aged 1 to 8 years old. (male, female)*
mtoto ambaye hajazaliwa dhiki	**fetal distress** *Term used to describe an abnormal heart rate or rhythm in a fetus indicating the need for urgent childbirth.*
mtoto ambaye hajazaliwa harakati	**fetal movements** *Sensations by the mother of fetal activity.*
mtoto ambaye hajazaliwa nafasi ndani ya mfuko wa uzazi	**fetal position** *Refers to how the fetus lies within the uterus.*
mtoto anayezaliwa akiwa mfu	**stillborn** *Refers to a newborn that died in utero.*
mtoto wa jicho	**cataract** *An opacity of an eye lens or the capsule.*
mtoto-wadogo	**baby-scale** *A device used to weigh an infant.*
mtu aliye kiziwi na bubu	**deaf-mute** *Inability to hear or speak.*
mtulinga	**clavicle** *A bone that articulates with the sternum and scapula.*
mtulinga	**collarbone** *Common term for the clavicle.*

Swahili	English
muda	**interval** *An intervening time.*
muda kabla ya kujifungua	**antenatal** *Refers to events before birth.*
muda kaimu	**long-acting** *Referring to a drug with long lasting effects.*
muda mrefu	**long-standing** *Having existed for a long time.*
muda mrefu wenye kuona	**longsighted** *Synonym of hyperopia.*
mufua	**cold** *Viral upper respiratory tract infection.*
muhimu	**essential** *Crucial or necessary.*
muhina	**nosebleed** *Common term for epistaxis.*
muhina; damu inapotoka kwenye pua	**epistaxis** *Bleeding emanating from the nose.*
mumuyika	**friable** *Easily reduced to powder.*
muongo	**decade** *Ten years.*
muundi	**shin** *Refers to the anterior tibial region.*
mvumo sikioni	**ringing in the ears** *Common term for tinnitus.*
mvumo sikioni	**tinnitus** *Medical term for ringing in the ears. It is associated with Meniere's syndrome among other conditions.*
mvungo wa wayo	**instep** *The medial aspect of the foot between the ankle and the ball of the foot.*
mvungu	**cavity** *Pouch or chamber.*
mvungu	**fossa** *A shallow depression.*
mvunjiko ambapo, mfupa umepondwa au kuvunjika kabisa	**fracture, comminuted** *A broken bone where one segment overrides the other.*
mvunjiko wa mfupa	**fracture** *A broken bone.*
mwaguzi; nesi	**nurse** *A person trained to care for the sick.*
mwaka	**year** *A time period that covers 365 days.*
mwanamke	**female** *Feminine.*
mwanamume	**man** *Male human.*
mwananamke aliyezaa mara moja	**primipara** *A woman giving birth for the first time.*
mwanya	**cleavage** *A sharp division or demarcation.*
mwanya	**crevice** *A narrow opening.*
mwanya mkubwa upande wa chini wa kichwa ambapo uti wa mgongo hupitia	**foramen magnum** *The hole in the skull that the spinal cord passes through.*
mwanzo	**onset** *The beginning of an event.*
mwanzo wa kuzaa; pata uchungu wa kuzaa	**labor onset** *The time when a pregnant woman begins uterine contractions in the process of childbirth.*
mwayo	**yawn** *Opening one's mouth and inhaling deeply due to sleepiness/boredom*
mwendawazimu	**insane** *A term not used in formal medical evaluations that when used by a layperson means a serious mental illness.*
mwendo	**gait** *The way one walks.*
mwendo usio wa hiari	**involuntary movement** *Movement not controlled consciously.*
mwenendo wa ugonjwa	**pathogenesis** *The course of a disease.*
mwezi; hedhi	**menstruation** *Synonym of menses.*
mwili	**body** *The physical structure of a person.*
mwili nywele; {vuzi}	**hair (of body) {axillary and pubic hair}**

Swahili	English
mwili uso eneo	**body surface area** *Dubois formula is: (weight in kilograms)to the 0.425th power x (height in centimeters) to the 0.725th power x 0.007184.*
mwisho	**last** *Final.*
mwisho kumweka	**end point** *The last stage of a process.*
mwishoni mwa mufupa miwili ya miguuni pahali imechukua muundo wa muiringo	**malleolus** *A bony protrusion on medial and lateral aspect of each ankle.*
mzio	**allergy** *An immune response by the body to a compound it is hypersensitive to.*
mzizimo, baridi; kitapo	**chill** *Sensation of coldness.*
mzunguko	**frequency** *Rate of occurrence.*
mzunguko	**rotation** *Movement around an axis.*
na kuangalia kwa	**check for, to**
najisi	**rape** *Forced sexual relations.*
nasuri	**fistula** *An abnormal communication between two organs or an organ and the skin, as in rectovaginal fistula.*
nasuri ya haja kubwa	**anal fistula** *An opening in the skin that tracts to the anal canal thus causing some fecal material to leak from the opening in the skin.*
nawiri	**healthy** *In good health.*
ncha (mwishoni) ya bega	**scapula** *Medical term for the shoulder blade.*
ncha ya kidole cha mkono	**fingertip** *Distal aspect of a finger.*
ndani kupotoka ya gumba	**hallux varus** *Medial deviation of the great toe.*
ndani ya	**inside** *Inner part, center.*
ndani ya	**internal** *Situated on the inside.*
ndani ya fuvu	**intracranial** *Within the cranial vault.*
ndani ya joto la mwili; halijoto	**temperature** *The degree of internal heat in a person's body.*
ndani ya mfuko la uzazi	**intrauterine** *Within the uterus.*
ndani ya mfupa	**intraosseous** *Within a bone.*
ndani ya misuli	**intramuscular** *Within a muscle.*
ndani ya tumbo	**intraabdominal** *Within the abdominal cavity.*
ndani ya tumbo jipu	**intraabdominal abscess** *A collection of pus in the abdomen.*
ndani ya ubongo	**intracerebral** *Within the cerebrum.*
ndewe	**earlobe** *The soft, fleshy inferior portion of the pinna.*
ndezi	**drowsiness** *Sleepiness. (in swahili ndezi also means rat)*
ndezi	**laxity** *A description of a joint that is loose. (ndezi also means rat in Swahili)*
ndoa ushauri nasaha	**marital counseling** *Therapy aimed at marriage reconciliation.*
ndogo bakuli kutumika kushikilia matapishi	**emesis basin** *A small bowl used to catch vomitus.*
ndogo malengelenge ambayo yanaonyesha kaswende	**rupia** *A sign of tertiary syphilis in which there are bullae or vesicles formed on the skin that erupt and form crusts.*
ndogo uvimbe kwenye ukope	**meibomian cyst** *An enclosed fluid collection along a sebaceous gland of the eyelid.*
ndoto	**dream** *The thoughts or images occurring during sleep.*
ndugu (mdogo)	**sibling** *A brother or sister. (younger sibling)*
ndui	**smallpox** *Variola.*

166

Swahili	English
nematodi	**nematode** *An endoparasite belonging to the class of the Nemathelminthes including roundworms and threadworms.*
nematodi mdudu kwamba ni vimelea	**pinworm** *Common term for Enterobius vermincularis; a nematode worm that is a parasite.*
nena	**speech** *Oral articulation.*
nene na nata uthabiti	**viscous** *Having a thick, sticky consistency.*
nene nyeupe ukeni	**leukorrhea** *Thick white vaginal discharge.*
ng'ombe wazimu ugonjwa	**mad cow disease** *Bovine spongiform encephalopathy, a disease that cause cerebral degeneration exhibited by ataxia.*
ngiri	**hernia** *An abnormal bulge of bowel through muscle.*
ngono	**coitus** *Sexual intercourse between members of the opposite sex.*
ngozi	**skin** *Flesh.*
ngozi dalili za ugonjwa	**exanthema** *A rash that accompanies a disease or fever.*
ngozi jirani moyo	**pericardium** *The structure enclosing the heart which contains a fibrous outer layer and serous inner layer.*
ngozi kati ya kwa kifua na mapafu	**pleura** *The serous membrane lining each lung.*
ngozi kavu na utando wa kamasi	**xerosis** *Pathological dryness of the skin or mucous membranes.*
ngozi nyembamba inayofunika sehemu ya ndani ya macho	**conjunctiva** *The membrane that lines the eyelid.*
ngozi tatu zinazofunika ubongo na uti wa mgongo	**meningeal** *Referring to the dura mater, arachnoid and the pia mater.*
ngozi ya kwanza ya juu	**dermis** *The "true skin" that lies beneath the epidermis.*
ngozi ya nje	**epidermis** *The skin cells overlying the dermis.*
ngumi	**fist** *When a person has their fingers clenched tightly to the palm.*
ngumu	**hard** *Rigid or very firm.*
ngumu bega	**frozen shoulder** *Common term for adhesive capsulitis.*
nguvu	**strong** *Having the power to move heavy objects.*
nguvu au uwezo	**potency** *Strength or power.*
nguvu ipimwayo wakati moyo unapokuwa katika hali ya kusongana unapopiga	**systolic** *Referring to systole or that which occurs during systole.*
nguvu; uwezo	**strength** *Force, might or vigor.*
nguyu	**knuckles** *Metacarpophalangeal joints or finger joints when the fist is closed.*
nishai	**inebriation** *Intoxication with drugs or alcohol.*
njaa	**starvation** *Death related to starvation.*
njaaa	**hunger** *A sense of discomfort caused by a lack of food.*
nje	**external** *Outside of the body.*
nje kugeuka ya macho	**exotropia** *A type of strabismus that is characterized by the eyes turned outward.*
njia tofauti na kusafiri kwa ajili ya damu au maji ya	**shunt** *An alternate path for blood or fluid.*
njia ya kuingia	**access** *Means of entry.*
nta ya sikio	**cerumen** *Waxy substance found normally in the external ear canals.*
nta ya sikio	**wax** *Cerumen.*

167

Swahili	English
nuru	**light** *Illumination, bright.*
nusu	**half** *Divided in two.*
nusu ya maisha	**half-life** *The time a drug decreases its effect in half over time.*
nyama nyembamba kama mshipa inayounganisha mfupa kwa mwingine	**ligament** *A band of fibrous connective tissue that connects two bones or cartilage.*
nyamavu	**silent** *Absence of noise or no indication of something.*
nyembamba ya kitundu	**stenosis** *Narrowing of an orifice.*
nyembamba ya mfereji	**stricture** *A narrowing of a canal or duct.*
nyembemba na vungu ukucha wa kidole cha mkono;	**koilonychia** *Thin and concave fingernails.*
nyeusi kinyesi	**black stools** *Common term for melena.*
nyoka (sumu ya nyoka)	**snake (snake venom)**
nyonga	**hip** *The lateral eminence of the pelvis from the waist to the thigh; it is formed by the iliac crest and greater trochanter.*
nyongea; chirwa	**rickets** *A condition exhibited by softening and bowing of the long bones; caused by Vitamin D deficiency.*
nyongeza	**accessory** *Complimentary or concomitant.*
nyongeza athari	**cumulative effect** *A consequence of successive additions.*
nyongo	**bile** *An alkaline fluid secreted by the liver to aid digestion.*
nyonyesha	**suckle, to** *An infant taking to his mother's nipple.*
nyuki	**bee sting** *A piercing from a bee.*
nyuma	**posterior** *Further back in position; opposite of anterior.*
nyuma harakati	**retrograde** *Referring to backward movement.*
nyuma harakati ya damu katika moyo (1) cheu (2)	**regurgitation** *1. Backflow of blood in the heart. 2. Movement of gastric contents into the mouth.*
nyuma sehemu ya mfupa kidunia	**mastoid** *Referring to the mastoid process.*
nyuma sehemu ya ubongo	**cerebellum** *The part of the brain in the posterior portion of the skull that controls muscle coordination and movement.*
nyungunyungu	**athlete's foot** *Common term for tinea pedis.*
nyungunyungu	**tinea pedis** *Ringworm of the feet, a fungal infection.*
nyutrofili	**neutrophil** *A polymorphonuclear leukocyte.*
nywele juu ya kichwa {udevu}	**hair (of head) {facial hair- beard}**
nywele juu ya ukope	**eyelash** *Each of the short hairs on the eyelid.*
nywele kupotea	**alopecia** *The absence of hair in areas where it normally exists.*
nywele kuruwili	**hirsutism** *Abnormal growth on hair on a person's face and body.*
nywele nyingi ukuaji	**hypertrichosis** *Excessive hair growth.*
nzito	**heavy** *Possessing great weight.*
nzuri karibu maono	**myopia** *Nearsightedness.*
oksijeni	**oxygen** *A colorless, odorless gas with atomic number 8.*
ondoka kitandani	**get up out of bed**
orodha ya ugunduzi inawezekana	**differential diagnosis** *A list of possible alternative diagnoses for a patient who is ill.*
ovundo	**odiferous** *Having an unpleasant or distinctive smell.*
pacha (pacha fanani)	**twins** *Two infants born at the same birthing.(identical twins)*
pafu	**lung** *One of a pair of respiratory organs.*

168

Swahili	English
pahali kidole cha mkono kinashikana na mkono	**metacarpophalangeal** *Referring to the metacarpus and the phalanges.*
pahali ndani ya chembechembe ambapo chckula huchomwa na kubadirishwa kuwa nguvu	**mitochondria** *Organelle found in cells responsible for energy production.*
paja	**thigh** *The body region between the inguinal crease and knee.*
paji la uso ni sehemu kuwasilisha wakati anapozaliwa	**brow presentation** *The term used to describe which part of the body (forehead) is being delivered first in childbirth.*
pamba	**cotton wool** *Raw cotton.*
pande; rugurugu	**lump** *A protuberance.*
pandikiza	**graft** *A piece of tissue surgically transplanted.*
panja	**temple** *The temporal fossa superior to the zygomatic arch.*
panua	**dilatation** *The process of becoming wider or larger.*
panya	**rat** *A rodent that looks like a large mouse.*
panya	**rodent** *A gnawing mammal that includes rats and mice.*
papatika	**flutter** *Used to describe a cardiac rhythm disturbance, as in atrial flutter.*
papo hapo	**acute** *Abrupt onset.*
pasipo kichwa	**acephalous** *A absence of a head.*
pasuka	**tear** *As in a vaginal tear after childbirth.*
pata kitanda	**admission (to hospital)** *To be admitted.*
pata nafuu; pona	**feel better or get better** *To have improved health symptomatically.*
payo	**delirium** *An acute mental state exhibited by altered thought processes and restlessness.*
payo mitikisiko	**delirium tremens** *A condition seen when alcohol is withdrawn which is exhibited by restlessness, hallucinations and tremors.*
pembeni	**peripheral** *Referring to an outward part or surface.*
penga kamasi	**nose, blow the**
pengo	**gaping** *Wide open.*
pepopunda	**tetanus** *A condition caused by Clostridium tetani which produces spasm and rigidity of voluntary muscles.*
pepopunda	**trismus** *Commonly called lockjaw, it is a spasm of the muscles supplied by the trigeminal nerve and is an early symptom of tetanus.*
perema; matubwitubwi; machapwi	**mumps** *A contagious viral disease that is exhibited by parotid swelling and puts males at risk for sterility. Also called epidemic parotitis.*
pia magoti	**kneeling** *Being on one's knees as in the prayer position.*
pia ya goti; kilegesambwa	**patella** *The bone situated in the anterior portion of the knee.*
pia ya mguu; kilegesambwa	**kneecap** *Common term for patella.*
piga chafya (chafya)	**sneeze, to** *To suddenly expel air from the nose and mouth because of nasal irritation. (a sneeze)*
piga chenga	**dribble, to** *To slowly, drip-by-drip, release urine for example.*
piga kelele	**yell, to** *To speak in a loud tone.*
pigo la moyo	**heart beat** *A single contraction of the heart.*
pingamizi la kuhara	**anti-diarrheal** *Medication used to treat diarrhea.*
pingamizi la kutapika	**antiemetic** *A medication used to control nausea.*

169

Swahili	English
pingili ya mgongo	**vertebra** *A term for each bone surrounding the spine.*
pisha hewa safi	**ventilation** *The movement of air into the lungs; generally meant to suggest by an artificial process.*
plasta	**cast; plaster cast** *Use of plaster of paris to immobilize an extremity.*
plasta	**plaster cast** *Use of gypsum impregnated gauze to immobilize fractured extremities.*
Pneumocystis nimonia	**pneumocystis jiroveci pneumonia.** *A pulmonary infection associated with AIDS. Formerly called pneumocystis carinii pneumonia*
poa	**cool** *Chilly or cold.*
polepole	**slow** *Unhurried.*
polepole, taratibu mwanzo	**insidious** *A slow, gradual and harmful advancement.*
pombe	**alcohol** *Ethanol or ethyl alcohol.*
pombe madawa ya kulevya	**alcoholism** *An addiction to alcohol.*
povu	**foam** *A mass of small bubbles in a liquid.*
povu	**froth** *Covered with a mass of small bubbles.*
povu kinywani	**froth at the mouth, to** *To have a mass of saliva with small bubbles in it coming out of the mouth.*
proteni isaidiayo kufanyika kwa vigaga au vidonge	**fibrin** *An insoluble protein formed when fibrinogen is acted upon by thrombin.*
proteni ngumu kwenye ngozi, kucha na nywele	**keratin** *A protein found in the skin, hair, nails and enamel of the teeth.*
protini	**protein** *A class of nitrogenous organic compound.*
pua	**nose** *The midface protuberance used for smelling and breathing.*
puma	**throb, to** *The beat with strong regular rhythm.*
pumbu; kende	**testicle** *One of a pair of organs in the male scrotum that produces sperm.*
pumu	**asthma** *An inflammatory disease of the lungs noteworthy because of reversible airway obstruction.*
pumzi	**breath** *One respiration.*
pumzi sauti	**breath sounds** *The noise heard upon auscultation with a stethoscope.*
punguza	**decline** *As in a decrease in status or health.*
punta	**running suture** *A method of sewing a wound in which there is a knot at each end and continuous otherwise.*
rahisi	**convenient** *Opportune or well-timed.*
rangi nyekundu ya damu	**hemoglobin** *An iron containing protein used for the transport of oxygen in blood.*
rangi nyeusi	**black** *Referring to the color, as in the color of coal.*
rangi ya buluu	**blue** *A color between green and violet.*
rangi ya kahawia	**brown** *Coffee-colored.*
rangi ya manjano	**yellow** *A color between green and orange in the spectrum*
riahi	**bloated** *Sensation of having an abnormally large amount of air in the viscera.*
riahi	**flatulence** *The gas expulsed from the anus.*
risasi na jeraha	**gunshot wound** *An penetrating injury sustained from a bullet.*

170

Swahili	English
rishai	**exudate** *The fluid, cells, and debris found in the tissues or a cavity (like pleural space) during inflammation.*
rosasia	**rosacea** *Erythema of the cheeks and nose caused by chronic vascular and follicular dilation.*
rovu; goita	**goiter** *Swelling of the thyroid gland.*
ruba la ini	**fluke** *Parasitic nematode worm; an example is Schistosoma.*
rubela	**rubella** *Also called German measles, it is characterized by a rash, fever, headache.*
sababu haijulikani	**idiopathic** *Relating to a disease with an unknown cause.*
sabuni	**soap** *A compound made with fats/oils and an alkali; it is used for washing.*
sahihi	**right** *Correct, accurate (adjective)*
sainosisi	**cyanosis** *Bluish discoloration of the skin and mucous membranes.*
sambamba	**compatible** *To coexist without problems.*
samtidiga	**simultaneous** *Occurring at the same time.*
saratani ya korodani	**seminoma** *A malignant tumor of the testis.*
sasa	**currently** *Presently.*
sauti	**voice** *The sound produced through the larynx and out the mouth.*
sauti za juu zinazotokana na kufinyika kwa njia za hewa	**stridor** *An abnormal, high-pitched, musical sound caused by an obstruction in the larynx or stenosis of the vocal cords.*
sawa	**analogous** *To resemble or be similar to.*
sawa	**equal** *The same or uniform.*
sawa	**right** *Sure, agreed, OK (adverb)*
sehemu laini katikati ya jino yenye hisia na mishipa ya damu	**pulp** *The tissue filling the root canals of a tooth.*
sehemu ya ndani ya ngozi ifunikayo ubongo na uti wa mgongo	**pia mater** *The first layer of three covering the brain and spinal cord.*
sehemu inayotokeza	**promontory** *A protruding eminence.*
sehemu kati ya kuma na mkundu	**perineal** *Referring to the perineum.*
sehemu nyembamba inayojitokeza kwenye kifupa cha pili cha uti wa mgongo ambapo kifupa cha kwanza cha uti wa mgongo huzungukia	**odontoid** *A prominence on the second cervical vertebra on which the first cervical vertebra pivots.*
sehemu nyembamba upande wa juu kwenye mfupa mkubwa wa mkono kati ya kiko na kiwiko	**olecranon** *The bony protrusion at the proximal ulna at the elbow.*
sehemu nyeupe ya mboni	**sclera** *The white outer covering of the eyeball.*
sehemu ya chini iliyo nyembamba katika chungu cha mtoto	**cervix uteri** *The narrow end of the uterus.*
sehemu ya chini ya mfupa wa kidari	**xiphoid process** *The inferior segment of the sternum.*

171

Swahili	English
sehemu ya kichimo kilicho nyuma ya pua, kinywa na kikoromeyo kati ya kaakaa laini na ulimi mdogo	**oropharynx** *The portion of the pharynx between the soft palate and the superior aspect of the epiglottis.*
sehemu ya kishimo kilicho nyuma ya pua, kinywa na kikoromeo juu ya kaakaa laini	**nasopharynx** *The part of the pharynx which lies superior to the soft palate*
sehemu ya mbele ya tegu	**scolex** *The front end of a tapeworm.*
sehemu ya nje ya sikio	**auricle** *The external portion of the ear.*
sehemu ya nyuma	**dorsal** *Referring to the back or back surface.*
sehemu ya ubongo ambayo huzimamia baadhi ya kazi za mwili kama urekebishaji wa joto	**hypothalamus** *Located inferior to the thalamus it controls visceral activities, water balance, temperature and sleep.*
sehemu ya ubongo inayounganisha ubongo na uti wa mgongo	**brain stem** *An organ that consists of the medulla oblongata, pons and midbrain.*
sehemu ya uu ya kila nusu ya moyo	**atrium** *Referring to a chamber used as an entrance, as in the entrance to the heart.*
sehemu yenye maji katika damu	**serum** *The fluid that isolates out when blood coagulates.*
sehemu yoyote ya tegu	**proglottis** *Any segment of a tapeworm.*
seli nyekundu za damu	**erythrocyte** *Called a red blood cell, it transports oxygen and carbon dioxide to and from the tissues.*
seli nyeupe ya damu	**leukocyte** *A white blood cell.*
selidamu	**blood cells** *A common term that does not differentiate between erythrocyte or leukocyte.*
sema tirivyogo	**mumble, to** *To speak quietly and indistinctly.*
senta	**concentric** *Referring to circles or arcs that share the same center.*
shaghala	**at random** *Occurring by chance alone.*
shashi ya pamba	**gauze** *A fabric used for dressing changes.*
shashi ya pamba	**swab** *An absorbent material used for cleaning wounds or applying ointment.*
shavu	**buccal** *Referring to the cheek.*
shavu	**cheek** *Lateral facial tissue.*
shavu la mguu	**calf** *Muscles of the posterior portion of the lower leg.*
shavu la mguu	**muscle, calf**
shavu la mkono	**muscle, biceps**
shida kumeza	**dysphagia** *Difficulty in swallowing.*
shingo	**neck** *The part of the body that connects the body to the head.*
shinikizadamu	**hypertension** *Higher than normal blood pressure.*
shinikizo la damu	**high blood pressure** *Elevated arterial blood pressure.*
Shirika la Afya Duniani	**World Health Organization (WHO)**
shituko harakati ya mikono	**asterixis** *Commonly known as a flapping tremor, it is characterized by involuntary jerking movements of the hands and is seen commonly in hepatic encephalopathy.*
shoti	**gallop** *An abnormal heart sound.*
shoto	**left-handed** *The preference of using the left hand for common tasks.*

172

Swahili	English
shtuko cha misuli usoni	**tic** *Periodic spasmodic facial muscle contractions.*
shuka ya kitanda	**sheet (bed)** *A rectangular fabric covering a bed.*
shuzi	**flatus** *Term for air that is expelled from the anus.*
si inatarajiwa	**unexpected** *Unforeseen.*
si kamili kupooza	**paresis** *Incomplete paralysis.*
si kukusudia haja kubwa	**encopresis** *Involuntary defecation.*
si kukusudia kukojoa	**enuresis** *Involuntary urination.*
si kwa hiari misuli kipindupindu ya zoloto	**laryngospasm** *Sudden, involuntary muscle contraction of the larynx.*
si ndoa	**single** *Not married.*
si rahisi kwa mara	**stiff** *Not easily bent.*
si rutuba (1), kuzaa	**sterile** *1. Infertile 2. Refers to equipment that is free of contamination.*
si wazi hotuba	**inarticulate** *Indistinct speech.*
sifongo kutumika katika upasuaji	**sponge** *Sterile fabric used to soak up fluid during surgery.*
sifuri	**zero** *No quantity.*
sikadiani	**circadian** *Referring to a 24 hour period.*
sikio	**ear** *The organ of hearing and balance.*
sikio la ndani	**ear, inner** *Auris interna.*
sikio maambukizi	**ear infection** *General term referring to otitis media or otitis externa.*
sikio mfereji imefungwa na nta	**cerumen impaction** *External ear canal full of wax resulting in hearing loss until the impaction is removed.*
sikitiko; masikitiko; sijiko	**sadness** *The state of being sad.*
sikitiko; msiba; buka	**sound** *Vibrations that travel through air and are heard when reaching the ears.*
simama	**stand** *To stop or to be upright*
sindano	**needle** *The slender cylindrical device attached to a syringe.*
sindano (choma sindano)	**injection** *The act of a needle being inserted into a body. (given injection)*
sindano ya maji katika mshipa	**infusion** *The injection of fluid into tissue or a vein.*
sindano; sirinji	**syringe** *A device used for administering medication through various routes.*
sisimka	**tingling** *Prickling or stinging sensation.*
sita kipindi cha wiki baada ya kujifungua	**puerperium** *The six week period after childbirth.*
sodo; usafi kitambaa	**feminine pad** *Gauze specially designed to absorb menstrual flow.*
sodo; usafi kitambaa	**sanitary napkin** *Cloth or synthetic material used to absorb menstrual blood.*
sogeza kwa upande	**abduct** *To move a body part away from the body.*
soksi	**socks** *Worn on the feet before one puts on shoes.*
songo harakati cha mikono	**athetosis** *An involuntary symptom exhibited by continuous slow, writhing movements, mostly in the hands.*
sotoka	**rinderpest** *A viral disease primarily of cattle that is thought to have been eradicated as of 2001.*

Swahili	English
sufuria kitanda	**bedpan** *A metal or plastic vestibule one sits on while in bed to defecate.*
sugu	**callosity** *Callus; thickened hardened skin.*
sukari	**sugar** *A sweet crystalline substance made from a plant such as sugar cane.*
sukari katika mkojo	**glycosuria** *Presence of glucose in the urine.*
sumaku	**magnet** *A piece of iron with atoms ordered to make it magnetic.*
sumu	**poison** *A substance that causes illness or death.*
sumu kwenye damu	**septicemia** *A systemic disease in which microorganisms or their toxins are in the blood stream.*
sumu monoksidi kaboni	**carbon monoxide poisoning** *This tasteless, odorless gas causes constitutional symptoms but can lead to death upon inhalation.*
sumu tindikali (plumbi)	**lead poisoning** *The ingestion of lead, exhibited in severe cases by paralysis, encephalopathy, purple gingiva, and colic.*
sumu ya nyoka	**venom (snake)** *A term used to describe the toxin injected via a bite or sting.*
sumu; liga	**toxin** *A poison of plant or animal origin.*
surua; ukambi	**measles** *A childhood viral, infectious disease exhibited by rash and fever.*
tabaka	**layer** *A stratum or thickness.*
tabia machafuko	**behavior disorder** *An abnormal mental state.*
tahadhari	**alert** *Being in a watchful, ready state.*
tako kuzaliwa	**breech birth** *Delivery with the feet or buttocks coming first.*
takriban	**approximately** *Nearly but not completely.*
tamaa	**craving** *An unusually strong urge for something.*
tamaa kubwa ya ulevi	**dipsomania** *Compulsion to drink alcoholic beverages.*
tangu kuzaliwa	**congenital** *A disease or anomaly present from birth.*
tangu kuzaliwa kaswende	**congenital syphilis** *Passed to the child in utero, the child may have failure to thrive, fever and a flattened bridge of the nose.*
tangu kuzaliwa, hali ya sifa kwa kuwa na vidole zaidi ya tano kwa upande mmoja	**polydactyly** *Congenital anomaly exhibited by more than 5 digits on the hands and/or feet.*
taratibu	**hydration** *Used to describe fluid balance.*
tarehe ya kuingia hospitalini	**date of admission** *Beginning date of hospitalization.*
tarehe ya kumalizika muda	**expiration date** *The date when a medication should no longer be used.*
tarehe ya kuondoka hospitali	**discharge date** *The day a patient is released from the hospital.*
tarehe ya kuzaliwa	**date of birth**
tarhe ya mwisho	**deadline** *Cutoff date.*
tathmini	**evaluation** *Assessment or evaluation.*
tatizo unasababishwa na matibabu	**iatrogenic** *A problem caused by medical treatment.*
tatu cheyo	**wisdom tooth** *Third molar.*
tauni ya majipu	**bubonic plague** *A form of plague exhibited by the formation of buboes.*
taya	**jaw** *Mandible.*
taya la chini	**mandible** *The lower jaw.*
tegu	**tapeworm** *A parasitic, intestinal flatworm.*

174

Swahili	English
tekekuwanga	**chicken pox, varicella** *A viral disease characterized by extremely pruritus blisters over the entire body.*
tekenya	**tickle, to** *To lightly touch a person to cause one to laugh.*
tekenywa	**chigger** *A parasitic mite of the genus Trombicula.*
teketeke	**flaccid** *Limp. A term applied to an extremity one cannot move actively.*
tembe	**capsule** *Medication in the form of a capsule.*
tembe; dawa; vidonge	**medication** *A substance used for medical treatment.*
tembe; dawa; vidonge	**medicine** *A substance used for medical treatment or the art and science of healing patients.*
tembe; dawa; vidonge	**pill** *A medicated tablet or capsule.*
tembe; dawa; vidonge	**tablet** *A small disk of a compressed solid substance.*
tetekuwanga	**varicella** *A virus that causes chickenpox and shingles. Also called herpes zoster.*
tetemeko	**tremor** *Involuntary contraction and relaxation of small muscle groups.*
tetemeko alibainisha wakati wa harakati, si katika mapumziko	**intention tremor** *The tremulous movement noted when a person is beginning to perform a task but not seen at rest.*
tezi	**tumor** *A benign or malignant overgrowth of tissue.*
tezi cha koo	**tonsil** *A rounded mass of lymphoid tissue, most commonly referring to the pharyngeal tonsil.*
tezi kibofu	**prostate** *A gland found in men that surrounds the neck of the urethra and bladder.*
tezi na kororo	**Graves' disease** *A form of hyperthyroidism exhibited by a goiter and exophthalmos.*
tezi ya kikoromeo	**thyroid** *A gland in the neck that secretes hormones regulating metabolism.*
thabiti	**consistent** *Compatible with something or congruous with.*
tiba	**curative** *A remedy capable of healing completely.*
tiba ya kuzuia maradhi	**prophylaxis** *That which is done to prevent disease.*
tiba ya mwili	**physical therapy** *Treatment of disease by heat, massage and exercise as opposed to medications.*
tibakemikali	**chemotherapy** *Use of medication (chemical agents) in the treatment of disease. This term is commonly used to refer to the treatment of cancer patients with medication.*
tibiwa	**treat, to** *Medical care one receives for illness or injury.*
tindikali	**lead** *An element with an atomic number of 82.*
tishu sampuli kwa kutumia sindano	**needle biopsy** *Use of a needle to aspirate body contents for microscopic or pathologic examination.*
tofauti na tofauti	**discrete** *Separate and distinct.*
tohara; tahiri	**circumcision** *Surgical excision of the foreskin.*
tojo	**tattoo** *A design made by inserting indelible ink into the skin.*
tokoni	**ilium** *The large bone at the superior aspect of the pelvis which is present bilaterally.*
tokwa na damu	**bleed** *Loss of blood.*
tokwa na jasho	**sweat, to** *The action of releasing moisture through pores of the skin.*
tone	**drop** *A single bit of fluid as in a drop seen while giving IV fluids.*

175

Swahili	English
towashi	**eunuch** *A man who has been castrated.*
tukio (matukio); ajali	**accident**
tumbo	**abdomen** *The portion of the body bordered by the diaphragm and the pelvis.*
tumbo	**stomach** *Organ of digestion between the esophagus and small bowel.*
tumbo kiwiliwili	**abdominal girth** *Waist circumference.*
tumbo la kuhara	**dysentery** *A severe form of diarrhea with blood and mucous in the stool.*
tumbo, upande wa juu	**epigastrium** *The section of the abdomen that overlies the stomach.*
tumbuka	**burst, to** *To rupture.*
tunaugua	**groan** *A deep inarticulate sound made due to pain or despair.*
tunda la pua	**nostril** *One of two openings in the nose used for air passage.*
tundu (tundu la jicho)	**socket** *An anatomical hollow that is part of an articulation. (eyeball socket)*
tundu katika mfupa	**foramen** *An opening in a bone.*
tunga usaha	**fester, to** *To become infected.*
tunga usaha	**suppuration** *Formation of purulent material.*
tupu	**empty** *Containing nothing.*
ubalehe	**puberty** *The time when adolescents become capable of sexual reproduction.*
ubaridi	**apathy** *Lack of interest in one's environment or indifference.*
uboho	**bone marrow** *The soft material filling the cavity of bones.*
ubongo	**brain** *A common term for cerebrum.*
ubongo kifu	**brain death** *Cessation of cerebral functioning.*
ubongo na uti wa mgongo	**central nervous system (CNS)** *The brain and spinal cord.*
uchaguzi	**choice** *Selection or decision.*
uchakacho	**hoarse** *A rough, harsh sounding voice.*
uchambuzi wa shahawa	**semen analysis** *Evaluation of semen used as part of a fertility workup.*
uchanga	**infancy** *Early childhood.*
uchokozi	**aggression** *Violent or hostile behavior.*
uchovu	**fatigue** *Tiredness and exhaustion.*
uchovu	**lethargy** *Absence of energy.*
uchovu	**tired** *Fatigued.*
uchovu; kujisikia vibaya	**malaise** *A vague feeling of discomfort or unease.*
uchungu wa kuzaa	**labor pains** *The intermittent pain associated with uterine contractions.*
uchunguzi	**screening** *An evaluation as part of a methodical study.*
uchunguzi baada ya kifo	**autopsy** *Examination of a body post-mortem in an attempt to determine cause of death.*
uchunguzi baada ya kifo	**necropsy** *Synonym of autopsy.*
uchunguzi upasuaji wa tumbo	**exploratory laparotomy** *Abdominal surgery with the intent of examining the abdominal contents.*
uchunguzi wa afya	**physical exam** *Examination of a client to assess their medical status.*
uchunguzi wa maabara	**laboratory test**

Swahili	English
udaifu unaoathiri upande mmoja wa mwili	**hemiparesis** *Unilateral muscle weakness (half the body).*
udanganyifu	**delusion** *A belief that is contradictory to rational thought.*
udhaifu	**debility** *Physical weakness.*
udhaifu	**weakness** *Feebleness.*
udhaifu unaotokana na kupoteza maji kwa ajili ya kutokwa na jasho kupita kiasa	**heat exhaustion** *A condition that occurs secondary to prolonged exposure to high ambient temperature; it is exhibited by subnormal temperature, dizziness and nausea.*
udhaifu wa misuli	**muscle weakness** *Decreased muscular function.*
udhaifu wa mwili	**asthenia** *Diminished strength and energy.*
udhaifu ya ukope	**ptosis** *Drooping of the upper eyelid usually due to paralysis of the third cranial nerve.*
udhibiti wa damu	**hemostasis** *The control of bleeding.*
uelewa	**empathy** *To be concerned for and share the feelings of another.*
ufa; mpasuko	**fissure** *A general term for a cleft or deep groove. An anal fissure, for example, is a small ulcer adjacent to the anus.*
ufahamu	**comprehension** *Understanding.*
ufanisi	**efficacious** *Effective.*
ufanisi	**ineffective** *Unsuccessful or inefficient.*
ufizi	**gingival** *Referring to the gums.*
ufizi	**gum** *Gingiva.*
ugiligili ya ubongo na uti wa mgongo (kuzunguka ubongo na uti wa mgongo)	**cerebrospinal fluid (CSF)** *The fluid between the pia mater and arachnoid membrane.*
ugiligili ya viungo (katika viungo kati ya mifupa)	**synovial fluid** *The fluid that surrounds, for example, the knee within a capsule.*
ugolo	**snuff** *Chewing tobacco.*
ugonjwa	**sickness** *Illness or a state of disease.*
ugonjwa kwamba itasababisha kifo	**terminal illness** *A disease with no viable treatment with death being inevitable.*
ugonjwa matokeo	**disease outcome** *The response obtained from treatment.*
ugonjwa mwendo	**motion sickness** *Nausea associated with travel.*
ugonjwa sifa kwa homa, kichefuchefu na upele	**rat bite fever** *As the name implies, it is a condition exhibited by fever, nausea and skin erythema after one is bitten by a rat.*
ugonjwa sifa kwa shingo ugumu, homa, na wakati mwingine kukosa fahamu	**meningitis** *Inflammation of the meninges exhibited by fever, photophobia, nuchal rigidity and in severe cases coma and convulsions.*
ugonjwa sifa kwa vipindi ya kukoma kinga wakati wa kulala	**sleep apnea** *Episodic apnea during sleep that is exhibited by daytime symptoms of fatigue, difficulty concentrating and sleepiness.*
ugonjwa ulioonyeshwa na kiu kubwa sana na mkojo	**diabetes insipidus** *Caused by a deficiency in vasopressin, it is exhibited by great thirst and large volume urine output (and normal blood sugar).*
ugonjwa unaoambukiza kwa njia ya kulalana	**sexually transmitted disease (STD)** *A condition one obtains from another during sexual relations.*
ugonjwa unaosababishwa na fangasi	**mycosis** *A disease caused by a fungal infection.*

177

Swahili	English
ugonjwa unaosababishwa na kula nyama ya kuambukizwa, ulioonyeshwa na homa na ugonjwa wa tumbo	**trichinosis** *A disease caused by meat infected by Trichinella spiralis causing fever and gastrointestinal effects.*
ugonjwa wa	**disorder** *Impairment.*
ugonjwa wa akilini kutokana na kupanda juu mlimani	**high altitude cerebral edema**
ugonjwa wa Alzheimer	**Alzheimer's disease** *A dementia of unknown cause or pathogenesis.*
ugonjwa wa asubuhi (kichefuchefu yanayohusiana na mimba)	**morning sickness** *Nausea associated with pregnancy.*
ugonjwa wa Crohn	**Crohn's disease** *An inflammatory bowel disease.*

178

Swahili-English: ugonjwa wa ini-zoloto

Swahili	English
ugonjwa wa ini	**cirrhosis** *A liver disease characterized by destruction of liver cells and increased connective tissue.*
ugonjwa wa kuambukiza	**infectious disease** *Any disease or condition considered contagious.*
ugonjwa wa kupooza	**paralysis** *Inability to move one or more extremities.*
ugonjwa wa mabaka ngozini	**hives** *Urticaria*
ugonjwa wa matezi	**adenopathy** *Generally referring to a condition of the lymphatic glands.*
ugonjwa wa midomo na miguu	**foot and mouth disease** *A contagious viral disease exhibited by oral and digital vesicles.*
ugonjwa wa sarufa, homa na upanuzi wengu unasababishwa na Leishmenia	**kala-azar** *A disease caused by Leishmania donovani that is exhibited by weight loss, fever, anemia and hepatosplenomegaly.*
ugonjwa wa sarufa, homa na upanuzi wengu unasababishwa na Leishmenia	**leishmaniasis** *A condition caused by a flagellate protozoan parasite that is exhibited by visceral or dermatologic manifestations.*
ugonjwa wa wanyama huambukizwa kwa binadamu	**zoonosis** *An animal-born disease that can be transmitted to humans, such as rabies.*
ugonjwa wa wanyama huambukizwa kwa binadamu	**zymogen** *An inactive compound that is metabolized to an active state.*
ugonjwa wa zinaa	**venereal disease** *A condition transmitted via sexual intercourse.*
ugonjwa ya sukari	**diabetes mellitus** *A disease exhibited by a deficiency of the pancreatic hormone insulin.*
ugua mifupa	**arthritis** *Joint inflammation.*
ugua mifupa na kisonono	**gonorrheal arthritis** *A type of arthritis caused by the gram negative diplococcus Neisseria gonorrhoeae.*
ugumu akizungumza	**dysarthria** *Difficulty in articulation of speech.*
ugumu akizungumza	**dysphasia** *Difficulty in speaking caused by cerebral dysfunction.*
ugumu au malalamiko	**problem** *Difficulty or complaint.*
ugumu au maumivu na kukojoa	**dysuria** *Difficulty or pain upon urination.*
uguza	**nursing care** *The assessment and treatment provided by nurses.*
uharaka	**urgency** *Emergency or priority.*
uhasi	**castration** *Excision of the gonads.*
uja uzito; mimba; himila	**pregnancy** *The period of being pregnant.*
ujana	**adolescence**
ujauzito	**gestation** *The development of a fetus from conception until birth.*
ujazi	**corpulence** *Fatness.*
ujumla	**general** *Common or expected.*
ujumla kuonekana	**general appearance** *The overall look of a patient.*
ukano	**tendon** *Fibrous tissue that connects muscle to bone.*
ukaushaji	**desiccation** *The act of drying up.*
ukaya wa ukucha	**cuticle** *The dead skin at the base of the toenail or fingernail, also called the eponychium.*

Swahili	English
uke	**vagina** *The canal in a female that extends from the vulva to the cervix.*
uke kinyaa	**discharge, vaginal** *Vaginal secretions.*
uke kinyaa (baada ya kujifungua)	**discharge, postpartum vaginal** *The secretions noted after delivery.*
ukimwi	**Acquired Immunodeficiency Syndrome (AIDS)** *Presence of an AIDS defining illness or having a CD4 of less than 200/mm3.*
UKIMWI	**AIDS** *Acquired Immunodeficiency Syndrome*
ukoma	**Hansen's disease** *Leprosy*
ukoma	**leprosy** *A contagious disease caused by Mycobacterium leprae that causes insensate papules and disfiguration.*
ukongwe	**old age** *A relative term for the period of advanced years.*
ukoo	**relation** *1. A person who has a blood or marriage connection.*
ukope	**eyelid** *Palpebra.*
ukope kuugeukia	**ectropion** *Eversion of the eyelid, usually the lower lid.*
ukosefu wa dalili	**asymptomatic** *The absence of symptoms.*
ukosefu wa harakati	**stasis** *Lack of movement.*
ukosefu wa hotuba ya kueleweka	**incoherent** *Absence of intelligible speech.*
ukosefu wa kinga mwilini	**immunodeficiency** *An inadequate immune response.*
ukosefu wa korodani	**anorchous** *The absence of testicles.*
ukosefu wa kula	**aphagia** *The lack of eating.*
ukosefu wa kupumua	**apnea** *Absence of respiration.*
ukosefu wa maambukizi ya	**asepsis** *Lack of infection.*
ukosefu wa maana ya ladha	**gustatory agnosia** *The loss of the sense of taste.*
ukosefu wa mkojo	**anuria** *The lack of urine excretion.*
ukosefu wa msawazo	**disequilibrium** *The absence of stability.*
ukosefu wa mzunguko wa hedhi	**amenorrhea** *The absence of menses.*
ukosefu wa shahawa	**aspermia** *Absence of sperm.*
ukosefu wa ubongo	**anencephaly** *The congenital absence of the cranial vault and cerebral hemispheres.*
ukosefu wa ufunguzi	**imperforate** *Lack of an opening. An infant with an imperforate anus has a congenital defect with no anal opening.*
ukosefu wa ulinganifu	**asymmetry** *Lack of symmetry.*
Ukosefu wa uratibu wa misuli	**ataxia** *Lack of muscular coordination.*
ukosefu wa uwezo wa harufu	**anosmia** *Lack of the sense of smell.*
ukosefu wa uwezo wa kiakili	**amentia** *The absence of mental ability.*
ukosefu wa uwezo wa kusema	**aphasia** *Diminished ability to communicate via speech or writing.*
ukosefu wa uwezo wa kusoma kutokana na ugonjwa wa ubongo	**alexia** *Inability to read due to a central brain lesion.*
ukosefu wa uwezo wa kutambua mambo au watu	**gnosia** *Ability to recognize things and people.*
ukosefu wa uwezo wa kutambua vitu ukoo	**anomia** *Inability to name or recognize familiar objects.*
ukosefuu wa mate	**aptyalism** *Diminished or absence of saliva.*
ukubwa	**size** *The dimensions of something.*

Swahili	English
ukucha	**nail** *The hard surface on the dorsal surface of the toes or fingers.*
ukucha wa kidole cha mguu	**toenail** *The nail at the tip/dorsal aspect of each toe.*
ukucha wa kidole cha mkono	**fingernail** *Thin horny plate over the dorsal aspect of the end of finger.*
ukungu	**fungus** *A spore-producing organism that feeds on organic matter.*
ukuruti	**itch** *A sensation that makes one want to scratch.*
ukurutu	**eczema** *A medical condition exhibited by pruritic, red, scaly patches on the scalp, cheeks and extensor surfaces.*
ukuta wa chungu cha mtoto	**endometrium** *The mucous membrane lining of the uterus.*
ukwanguaji	**curettage** *Removal of tissues from a cavity.*
ulaji	**diet** *The kinds of food a person eats.*
ulaji wa chakula	**food intake** *Quantitative record of nutritional intake.*
ulemavu wa miguu yote	**paraplegia** *Paralysis of the lower extremities.*
ulemavu wa mikono yote miwili na miguu yote	**quadriplegia** *Paralysis of all four extremities.*
ulemavu wa mkono mmoja au mguu	**monoplegia** *Paralysis of a single limb.*
ulemavu wa mwili nusu	**hemiplegia** *Paralysis of one side of the body.*
ulevi	**drunk** *Inebriated.*
ulevi na dhiki	**dual diagnosis** *Term used to describe the presence of alcohol/drug addiction associated with a psychiatric diagnosis such as depression.*
ulimi	**tongue** *The fleshy muscular organ of the mouth.*
ulinganifu	**symmetry** *Being equally bilaterally.*
uliopooza misuli	**atrophy** *A diminution in the size of a part.*
ulozi; uchawi	**sorcery** *Black magic or voodoo.*
uma	**sting** *A small puncture as in a bee sting.*
umbali kati ya vitu	**span** *A distance between two objects.*
umbo kama msalaba	**cruciform** *Shaped like a cross.*
umio ; umio wa chakula	**esophagus** *The muscular tube that connects the throat to the stomach.*
umio wa pumzi	**trachea** *The ringed canal between the pharynx and bronchi.*
umivu	**ache** *A mild pain*
umo la mdudu ngozini	**insect bite**
umri (umri mkubwa)	**age** *Length of life.(old age)*
umri-kuhusiana na kusikia hasara	**presbyacusia** *An age related, progressive hearing loss.*
umwagaji damu kinyesi	**hematochezia** *Presence of blood in the excrement.*
umwagaji damu kinyesi	**melena** *The passage of black, tarry stools indicative of upper gastrointestinal bleeding.*
unafuu	**relief** *Alleviation from pain or discomfort.*
Unaozidi	**increment** *An increase on a fixed scale.*
unene	**obesity** *Having a body mass index over 30kilograms/meters squared.*
unga dawa	**compound** *A substance formed by covalent union of two or more atoms.*

181

Swahili	English
unguza unaosababishwa na maji ya moto	**scald** *A burn injury from extremely hot water.*
unyamavu	**quiet** *Making little or no noise.*
unyanyasaji	**abuse (sexual abuse)**
unyevu	**moist** *Damp or humid.*
unyushi	**eyebrow** *Supercilium.*
uoga wa kutangamana na watu	**agoraphobia** *The fear of being in a large open space.*
uokoaji	**evacuation** *The emptying of an organ of fluids or gas.*
uondoaji	**withdrawal** *The action of being without drugs or alcohol.*
upana	**width** *Side to side measurement.*
upande	**lateral** *Referring to the side of the body.*
upande	**side** *A position medial or lateral to center.*
upande wa juu wa ngozi ifunikayo ubongona uti wa mgongo	**epidural** *The space around the dura of the spinal cord.*
upande wa mbele	**frontal** *Referring to the anterior aspect, as in frontal lobe.*
upande wa nje wa ngozi ifunikayo ubongo na uti wa mgongo	**dura mater** *The outermost covering of the brain and spinal cord.*
upande wa nyuma ya goti	**popliteal fossa** *The hollow in the posterior aspect of the knee joint.*
upando huo	**ipsilateral** *On the same side.*
upanuzi	**expansion** *Enlargement or increase in size.*
upanuzi wa ini	**hepatomegaly** *Enlargement of the liver.*
upanuzi wa mifupa ya miguu na mikono na uso	**acromegaly** *Hyperplasia of the nose, jaw, fingers and toes.*
upasuaji	**operation** *A surgical procedure.*
upasuaji akifanya kwenye pua	**rhinoplasty** *Plastic surgery performed on the nose.*
upasuaji badala ya konea	**corneal transplant** *Surgical replacement of a cornea with a donor cornea.*
upasuaji badala ya nyonga	**hip replacement** *Both joint surfaces are replaced by high density material such as plastic or metal.*
upasuaji chale ya kifua	**thoracotomy** *Surgical incision of the thorax.*
upasuaji chale ya sehemu nyeupe ya mboni	**sclerotomy** *Surgical incision of the sclera.*
upasuaji kanzu	**gown** *A sterile gown used during surgical procedures.*
upasuaji kuondoa kibole	**appendectomy** *Surgical excision of the appendix.*
upasuaji kuondoa nyongo	**cholecystectomy** *Surgical excision of the gallbladder.*
upasuaji kuondoa sehemu ya kaakaa	**pallidectomy** *Surgical resection of all or part of the palate.*
upasuaji kuondoa sehemu ya kongosho	**pancreatectomy** *Surgical excision of part or all of the pancreas.*
upasuaji kuondoa sehemu ya utumbo mdogo	**enterectomy** *Surgical resection of part of the intestine.*
upasuaji kuondoa wengu	**splenectomy** *Surgical excision of the spleen.*
upasuaji kuondolewa cha kilegesambwa	**patellectomy** *Surgical excision of the patella.*

Swahili	English
upasuaji kuondolewa cha koko	**orchidectomy** *Synonym of orchiectomy; removal of one or both testes.*
Upasuaji kuondolewa figo	**nephrectomy** *Surgical removal of a kidney.*
upasuaji kuondolewa kwa bawasiri	**hemorrhoidectomy** *Surgical excision of a hemorrhoid.*
upasuaji kuondolewa kwa ini	**hepatectomy** *Partial or complete surgical resection of the liver.*
upasuaji kuondolewa kwa jicho	**enucleation** *Surgical removal of a globe.*
upasuaji kuondolewa kwa jiwe figo	**nephrolithotomy** *Surgical removal of a renal calculus.*
upasuaji kuondolewa kwa kidaka tonge	**uvulectomy** *Excision of the uvula.*
upasuaji kuondolewa kwa mfuko wa uzazi	**hysterectomy** *Surgical removal of the uterus.*
upasuaji kuondolewa kwa mkono au mguu	**amputation** *Typically referring to the surgical removal of a limb.*
upasuaji kuondolewa kwa mrija kutoka figo na kibofu cha mkojo	**ureterectomy** *Surgical resection of one or both ureters.*
upasuaji kuondolewa kwa njia ya haja kubwa	**proctectomy** *Surgical excision of the rectum.*
upasuaji kuondolewa kwa ovari	**oophorectomy** *Surgical removal of an ovary.*
upasuaji kuondolewa kwa tumbo	**gastrectomy** *Complete or partial surgical resection of the stomach.*
upasuaji kuondolewa kwa ulimi	**glossectomy** *Surgical resection of the whole or part of the tongue.*
upasuaji kuondolewa matumbo kubwa	**colectomy** *Surgical removal of part of the colon.*
upasuaji kuondolewa moja au zote mbili matiti	**mastectomy** *Surgical resection of one or both breasts.*
upasuaji kuondolewa neva	**neurectomy** *Excision of a section of a nerve.*
upasuaji kuondolewa tezi kibofu	**prostatectomy** *Surgical excision of the prostate.*
upasuaji kuondolewa tezi ya kikoromeo	**thyroidectomy** *Surgical resection of all or part of the thyroid.*
upasuaji kuondolewa umio	**esophagectomy** *Surgical removal of the esophagus.*
upasuaji kuondolewa ya zoloto	**laryngectomy** *Surgical removal of the larynx.*
upasuaji kuondolewa yote au sehemu ya uvimbe	**pneumonectomy** *Surgical excision of all or part of a lung.*
upasuaji maalum ya mifupa	**orthopedics** *A surgical specialty concerned with treatment of skeletal problems.*
upasuaji matengenezo ya kiwambo cha sikio	**tympanoplasty** *Restoration of the tympanic membrane's continuity.*
upasuaji matengenezo ya mrija wa mkojo	**urethroplasty** *Surgical repair of the urethra.*
Upasuaji uhusiano kati ya vipande viwili tofauti za mwili	**anastomosis** *Surgical formation of a connection between two previously separate parts.*
upasuaji viumbe wa ufunguzi katika mfuko wa tumbo	**gastrostomy** *A surgical creation of an opening in the stomach.*
upasuaji viumbe wa ufunguzi katika umio wa pumzi	**tracheostomy** *Creation of a surgical opening in the trachea so a tube could be placed in the trachea.*

Swahili	English
upasuaji viumbe wa ufunguzi katika zoloto	**laryngotomy** *Surgical creation of an opening in the larynx.*
upasuaji wa kutoa mtoto	**cesarean section** *Incision of the abdominal and uterine walls in order to deliver a fetus when natural delivery is not possible.*
upasuaji wa kuwashirikisha fuvu	**craniotomy** *Surgical creation of a hole in the skull.*
upasuaji wa ngiri kukarabati	**herniorrhaphy** *The surgical repair of a hernia.*
upasuaji wa tumbo chale	**laparotomy** *A surgical incision of the abdomen.*
upasuaji wa ubongo au uti wa mgongo	**neurosurgery** *Surgery of the brain or spinal cord.*
upatikanaji	**availability** *A person or thing that is available.*
upele	**scabies** *A skin condition exhibited by intense pruritus and a macular rash commonly in the perineal and interdigital spaces.*
upele wa malengelenge	**impetigo**
upendeleo	**biased** *Prejudiced.*
upimaji	**examination** *Assessment or evaluation.*
upofu	**blindness** *Absence of visual perception.*
upofu wa usiku	**hemeralopia** *Night blindness.*
upofu wa usiku	**night blindness** *Common term for nyctalopia, it refers to low vision with reduced illumination, often seen with Vitamin A deficiency.*
uponyaji	**healing** *The process of becoming healthy again.*
upotevu	**disappearance** *An instance of something/someone gone missing.*
upungufu	**decrease** *Becoming smaller or fewer.*
upungufu	**deficiency** *Insufficiency or deficit.*
upungufu wa asidi nikotini ulioonyeshwa na kuhara na ugonjwa wa ngozi	**pellagra** *A deficiency in nicotinic acid exhibited by diarrhea and dermatitis.*
upungufu wa damu	**anemia** *Lower than normal red blood cell count.*
upungufu wa maji mwilini	**dehydration** *The status of having a decrease in total body water.*
urefu	**length** *The end to end measurement.*
urefu wa muda mtu anatarajiwa kuishi	**life expectancy** *The length of time a person is anticipated to live.*
usaha katika mkojo	**pyuria** *Presence of purulent material in the urine.*
usaha katika mvungu wa mwili, kawaida kifua	**empyema** *A collection of purulent material in a body cavity, usually referring to a thoracic empyema.*
usambazaji	**dissemination** *To be spread or dispersed widely.*
usambazaji	**distribution** *The manner in which something is shared or spread out.*
usiku	**nocturnal** *Referring to events that happen at night.*
usimamizi	**management** *The process of dealing with things or people.*
usingizi	**insomnia** *Sleeplessness.*
usingizi (usingizi mzito)	**sleep** *A nap or a snooze. (deep sleep)*
usingizi mfupi	**nap** *A brief sleep or catnap.*
usingizi-kutembea	**somnambulism** *Sleepwalking.*
usio wa kawaida	**atypical** *Not usual.*

184

Swahili	English
usiokuwa wa kawaida hofu ya maji	**hydrophobia** *Abnormal fear of water.*
usiokuwa wa kawaida jasho	**dyshidrosis** *Disregulation of sweating*
usiokuwa wa kawaida kuongezeka kwa unyeti	**hypersensitivity** *Abnormal increase in sensitivity.*
usiokuwa wa kawaida mbele ya hewa kati ya mapafu na ukuta kifua	**pneumothorax** *Abnormal presence of air between the lung and chest wall.*
usiokuwa wa kawaida misuli harakati	**dyskinesia** *Abnormal movement.*
usiokuwa wa kawaida mkusanyiko wa maji katika kifua	**hydrothorax** *Accumulation of fluid within the thoracic cavity.*
usiokuwa wa kawaida ongezeko katika mate	**polysialia** *Abnormal increase in saliva.*
usiokuwa wa kawaida shinikizo kutumiwa na uti wa mgongo	**cord compression** *Pressure being applied to the spinal cord.*
usiokuwa wa kawaida tabia ya kula	**eating disorder** *General term for pathologic eating habits.*
usiokuwa wa kawaida usikivu kwa mwanga	**photophobia** *Abnormal sensitivity to light.*
usiokuwa wa kawaida utvidgningen ya matumbo kubwa	**megacolon** *Abnormal enlargement and dilatation of the colon.*
usiokuwa wa kawaida utvidgningen ya wengu	**splenomegaly** *An abnormally enlarged spleen.*
usiokuwa wa kawaida uwepo wa damu katika kifua	**hemothorax** *The abnormal presence of blood in the pleural cavity.*
usiokuwa wa kawaida uwepo wa damu kuzunguka bitana ya moyo	**hemopericardium** *Abnormal presence of blood in the pericardium.*
uso	**face** *Anterior aspect of the head from the forehead to the chin.*
usuha	**pus** *Thick yellow or green opaque liquid as seen with infection.*
utafiti wa muundo wa mwili	**anatomy** *The study of body structure.*
utafiti wa wanyama	**zoology** *The study of animals.*
utambi	**peritoneum** *The serous membrane covering the abdominal organs and lining the abdominal walls. (utambi also means wick in Swahili)*
utambuzi	**cognition** *The process of acquiring thought or understanding.*
utapiamlo	**malnutrition** *Lack of appropriate nutrition.*
utapio mlo	**kwashiorkor** *A form of malnutrition from inadequate protein intake.*
utata	**contraindication** *A situation in which two elements are inconsistent.*
utata jinsia kitambulisho	**genital ambiguity** *A disorder of sexual development in which the genitalia are not sufficiently developed to tell clearly if the person is male or female.*
utawala wa damu ndani ya vena	**transfusion** *Administration of blood products intravenously.*
utegemezi wa dawa	**drug dependence** *Addiction to a substance.*
utekelezaji	**implementation** *The process of putting a plan into effect.*

Swahili	English
utezi	**appointment** *A previously scheduled time to see a person.*
uthubutu wa mwili baada ya kifo	**rigor mortis** *The normal stiffening of the muscles and joints that occurs a few hours after death.*
uti wa mgongo	**spinal cord** *The bundle of nerves that with the brain comprise the central nervous system.*
uti wa mgongo	**vertebral column** *The cervical, thoracic and lumbar vertebrae.*
utoaji wa maziwa	**lactation** *The secretion of milk from mammary glands.*
utongo	**eye discharge** *Conjunctival discharge.*
utosi	**fontanelle or fontanel** *The space between the bones in the skull that are separate at birth.*
utosi	**vertex** *The crown of the head.*
utoto	**childhood** *The time between infancy and puberty.*
utu	**personality** *Qualities that form a person's unique character.*
utvidgningen	**enlargement** *Becoming bigger.*
utvidgningen ya matiti	**gynecomastia** *Enlargement of the breasts.*
uume; mboo	**penis** *Male genital organ used for the transfer of sperm and elimination of urine.*
uundwaji wa ufunguzi upasuaji katika mfupa	**osteotomy** *Creation of a surgical opening in bone.*
uvimbe	**swelling** *An abnormal enlarged from fluid collection.*
uvimbe kuwa haina kuondoka anatengeneza	**nonpitting edema** *Subcutaneous swelling that cannot be indented with compression.*
uvimbe wa kibofu cha mkojo	**distension** *Swollen.*
uvimbe wa nyuzi	**cystic fibrosis** *A congenital disorder exhibited by abnormal thick mucous which leads to problems in the intestines, pancreas and lungs.*
uvimbemchu ngu wa kifuko	**torsion** *Refers to twisting. Testicular torsion is the twisting of the spermatic cord that can lead to ischemia and gangrene of the testicle.*
uvimbemchu ngu wa kifuko; kimio	**tonsillitis** *Inflammation of the tonsils.*
uviringo ya uume wakati simika	**Peyronie's disease** *Curvature of the penis during an erection due to plaque.*
uvumbi	**powder** *Fine dry particles.*
uvungu	**hollow** *An indentation.*
uvuzi	**pubic hair** *Hair present in the perineal area.*
uwati; upele	**rash** *Exanthema or urticaria.*
uwekaji wa maji katika mjiko	**enema** *A procedure involving insertion of fluid into the rectum.*
uwezekano	**likelihood** *The probability or feasibility.*
uwezo wa jicho kuzoea kuona tofauti katika umbali	**accommodation** *A term used to describe the ability of the eye to adjust to various distances.*
uwezo wa kuishi	**viable** *Referring to a fetus that can survive childbirth.*
uwezo wa kuona katika umbali mkubwa	**hyperopia** *Farsightedness.*
uwezo wa kutambua kitu kwa kugusa	**stereognosis** *The ability to identify an object by touch.*
uwezo wa kutumia mikono yote miwili kwa wepesi	**ambidextrous** *Ability to use both hands equal ability.*
uwezo wa kuzaa	**fertility** *The ability of a person to contribute to contraception.*

186

Swahili	English
uyoka; eksirei	**x-ray**
uzalishaji wa manii	**spermatogenesis** *The production of spermatozoa.*
uzalishaji ya machozi	**lacrimation** *The secretion of tears.*
uzazi	**birth** *The process of bearing offspring from the uterus.*
uzazi wa majira	**birth control** *Any method of limiting contraception.*
uzazi wa mpango	**contraceptive** *A device or medication used to prevent pregnancy.*
uzazi wa mpango	**family planning** *Birth control.*
uzazi wa mtoto	**childbirth** *Parturition; the process of labor and delivery of an infant.*
uzee	**senility** *The process of being senile.*
uzi wa kufungia kitovu	**umbilical tape** *Material used to tie off the umbilical cord prior to cutting it after the baby is born.*
uzimuaji	**dilution** *The process of making a weaker solution.*
uzingatiaji	**adherence** *To stick to something figuratively or literally.*
uzito wa akili	**stupor** *A reduced level of consciousness.*
uzito wa mwili	**body weight** *Relative mass as measured in kilograms or pounds.*
uziwi	**deafness** *Having impaired hearing.*
uzoevu; mraibu	**addiction** *An abnormal dependency.*
uzuiaji	**occlusion** *A pathway that is blocked or obstructed.*
vena	**vein** *A vessel carrying blood back toward the heart.*
vena ndogo	**ventriculography** *Roentgenography of the ventricles after administration of contrast media.*
vidonda tumbo; alasi	**stomach ulcer** *Gastric ulcer.*
vifaa	**supplies** *Stock or reserves.*
vijana	**young** *Having lived for a short period.*
vijidudu virusi	**HIV** *Abbreviation for human immunodeficiency virus.*
vilio	**clot** *A thrombus or embolus.*
vilio	**coagulation** *The formation of a clot.*
vilio la damu ngozini	**ecchymosis** *Skin discoloration caused by bleeding beneath the epidermis.*
vimelea mapafu maambukizi yanayosababishwa na kinyesi ndege	**histoplasmosis** *A fungal pulmonary infection from bat and bird excrement.*
vimelea wa magonjwa ya ukucha wa kidole cha mkono	**onychomycosis** *Fungal disease of the toenails or fingernails.*
vinavyolingana	**matching** *Corresponding in pattern or style.*
vinjia vidogo vya hewa kwenya mapufu	**bronchiole** *A small branch that a bronchus divides into.*
vipaji asili	**aptitude** *A natural talent for something.*
vipele ngozini	**skin rash** *Dermal exanthema.*
vipindi	**intermittent** *Occurring at irregular intervals.*
virusi maambukizi yanayoathiri pua kwa ndani	**rhinitis** *A viral infection or allergic reaction exhibited by nasal mucosal inflammation.*
vitanda	**beds** *A mattress resting on a frame. (plural)*

Swahili	English
vitu vinavyokaa kama vidole vya mkono mwishoni mwa mfereji wa fallopian	**fimbria** *A slender projection at the end of the fallopian tube near the ovary.*
viungo vya kutoa sauti na nafasi iliyo kati kati ya viungo hivyo	**glottis** *Essentially the vocal structure, including the true vocal cords and the opening between them.*
viungo vya ndani vya tumbo kama vinaonekana na kutokea nje baada ya kidonda wazi	**evisceration** *The removal of bowels from the body.*
viungo vya uzazi	**genitalia** *Genitals.*
viungo vya uzazi chunjua	**genital wart** *The common term for Condylomata acuminata.*
vuguvugu	**tepid** *Lukewarm.*
vuja kwa maji kutoka jeraha	**weep, to** *To ooze fluid, such as from a wound.*
vumbi	**dust** *Dry earthen particles found on the ground and surfaces.*
vunja chupa	**ruptured membranes** *Signal of onset of labor (in Swahili it is commonly called "break the bottle")*
vunja chupa kwa zaidi ya saa 24	**prolonged rupture of the membranes** *Rupture of the membranes more than 24 hours before delivery.*
vya tenganisho;	**septum** *A wall separating two chambers, the nasal septum for example.*
wachache zaidi ya tano vidole juu mkono	**oligodactyly** *Presence of fewer than 5 digits on a hand or foot.*
wafu mfupa katika mifupa awali kujeruhiwa	**sequestrum** *Necrotic bone present in an injured or diseased bone.*
wagonjwa mahututi	**intensive care** *Vigorous treatment of the acutely ill.*
wajawazito	**gravida** *Pregnant.*
wakati bavu mbili au zaidi zimevunjika katika sehemu mbili au zaidi na kuacha sehemu ya ubavu imeninginia	**flail chest** *The term used when one has multiple rib fractures causing a segment of the chest wall to move incongruently with the rest of the chest wall.*
wakati kanda ya kitovu inatoka kabla ya mtoto wakati wa kuzaliwa	**prolapse of the umbilical cord** *Refers to the umbilical cord protruding from the cervix during active labor.*
wakati mifupa inarudia uhusiano wa kawaida kila mfupa kitika sehemu yake	**reduction** *Return of a dislocated joint or fractured bone to its proper position.*
wakati ugonjwa ni kupatikana kwa kawaida katika idadi ya watu	**endemic** *When a disease is commonly found in a location or in a people group.*
wakati wa shughuli hakuna	**quiescent** *A time of inactivity.*
wakubwa	**older** *Being around more than compared with another.*
waliohifadhiwa	**frozen** *Past participle of to freeze. Freeze: turn a liquid into a solid.*
wanakuwa wamemaliza kuzaa	**menopause** *The time when menstruation ceases.*
wanaougua	**sigh** *A long deep exhalation that expresses an emotion, as in relief.*
wapole	**harmless** *Safe or benign.*
wasiwasi	**anxiety** *Nervousness or unease.*
wasiwasi	**apprehensive** *A fear that something unpleasant will happen.*
wasiwasi	**worry, to** *To fret or have unease.*
watazamaji tu	**passive** *Not achieved through active effort.*

Swahili	English
watoto (mtoto); mwana	**offspring** *One's children. (child)*
watoto wachanga	**infant** *Newborn.*
Watoto wachanga hadi nne umri wa wiki	**neonate** *The term for a newborn infant for the first four weeks.*
watoto wachanga waliozaliwa baada ya kipindi kirefu kuliko kawaida ujauzito	**post-term birth** *An infant born after the normal length of pregnancy.*
watoto watatu waliozaliwa mimba moja	**triplets** *Three infants born during one birth.*
watu wazima	**adult** *Generally considered a person over 18 years old.*
wayo	**foot (sole of the foot)** *The lower extremity distal to the ankle.*
wayo	**plantar** *Referring to the bottom of the foot.*
wayo	**sole of foot** *Common term for plantar aspect of the foot.*
wazee	**elderly** *Advanced in years.*
wazi	**clear** *Transparent.*
wazi moja wa koo	**clear one's throat, to** *To cough lightly in attempt to speak more clearly.*
wazimu	**dementia** *A chronic brain disorder exhibited by memory loss, personality changes and faulty reasoning.*
wazimu baada ya kujifungua	**postpartum psychosis** *A episode of abnormal thought or hallucinations following delivery.*
wazimu; kichaa	**madness** *Common term for insanity.*
wazimu; maruerue	**hallucination** *A perception that is not based on reality.*
waziwazi	**overt** *Not hidden.*
wengu; bandama	**spleen** *The visceral organ that is involved with production and removal of blood cells.*
wenye kuona mbali	**presbyopia** *Farsightedness associated with aging.*
weupe	**pallor** *Unusually pale appearance.*
wiani	**density** *The denseness of an object.*
wima	**upright** *Vertical or standing.*
wingi	**plethora** *An excess of something.*
within the umio wa pumzi	**endotracheal** *Within the trachea.*
yai kuachiliwa kutoka kwa kifuko cha mayai ndani ya tumbo la mwanamke	**ovulation** *The release of an ova from the ovary.*
yasiyo ya kawaida	**arrhythmia** *An abnormal heart rhythm.*
yenye nguvu; uzito mwingi	**hyperbaric** *Use of gas at a higher than normal pressure.*
yumba	**stagger, to** *To walk in an unsteady fashion.*
za mwili	**bilateral** *Referring to both sides.*
zahanati	**clinic** *A building where patients are evaluated.*
zaidi ya	**beyond** *On the farther side.*
zaidi ya mmoja kiraka ya akimosi	**purpura** *The presence of patches of ecchymosis or petechiae.*
zaidi ya mmoja kuishi kuzaliwa	**multipara** *A woman with more than one live births.*
zaliwa	**born, to be** *Being present as a result of birth.*
zamani	**former** *Prior.*
zambarau kubadilika rangi ya ngozi	**port-wine mark** *Also called nevus flammeus, it is a vascular anomaly characterized by purplish skin discoloration.*

Swahili	English
zana	**equipment** *Apparatus or instrument.*
zaweza kuepukwa	**avoidable** *That which can be stopped or inhibited.*
zeri	**balm** *A topical medical preparation.*
zeruzeru	**albino** *A person who lacks pigment in the eyes, skin and hair.*
ziada	**excess** *Surplus or overabundance.*
zilizopitwa na wakati	**outdated** *Something that has passed the expiration date.*
zimia; zirai	**fainting** *The act of losing consciousness.*
zinazotokea bila ya uchochezi	**spontaneous** *Occurring without provocation.*
zindiko	**antibody** *A protein that combines with and counteracts foreign substances.*
zingizi	**after-pains** *The pain experienced after childbirth caused by uterine contractions.*
zingizi	**menstrual cramps**
ziwa	**breast** *Mammary tissue including the areola.*
ziwi (kiziwi)	**deaf** *Absence of the sense of hearing. (deaf person)*
zoezi	**habit** *A custom or inclination.*
zoloto; kikoromeo	**larynx** *A hollow muscular structure that contains the vocal cords.*

Postscript

Made in the USA
San Bernardino, CA
13 September 2014